BIOTERRORISM

Field Guide to

Disease
Identification

and

Initial Patient
Management

BIOTERRORISM

Field Guide to

Disease Identification

and

Initial Patient Management

Dag K. J. E. von Lubitz

CRC PRESS

Boca Raton   London   New York   Washington, D.C.

Library of Congress Cataloging-in-Publication Data

von Lubitz, Dag K. J. E.
    Bioterrorism : field guide to disease identification and initial
patient management / Dag K.J.E. von Lubitz.
        p. cm.
Includes index.
    ISBN 0-8493-2030-5 (alk. paper)
    1. Bioterrorism—Handbooks, manuals, etc. 2. Communicable
diseases—Prevention—Handbooks, manuals, etc. 3. Emergency medical
services—Handbooks, manuals, etc. I. Title.
    RC88.9.T47V66 2003
    616.9—dc21   20030531

Visit the CRC Press Web site at www.crcpress.com

© 2004 by Dag K.J.E. von Lubitz

No claim to original U.S. Government works
International Standard Book Number 0-8493-2030-5
Library of Congress Card Number 20030531
Printed in the United States of America 1 2 3 4 5 6 7 8 9 0
Printed on acid-free paper

CONTENTS

PREFACE

The outbreak of anthrax infections that followed shortly after September 11, 2001 showed that while we can defend ourselves against bioterrorism, our defenses are inefficient and need rapid improvement. Probably the most prominent deficiency in our ability to swiftly counteract the terrorist use of biological weapons is the general unfamiliarity with the presentations of the relevant infectious diseases, their recognition, and treatment. It is precisely this knowledge that is fundamental to our ability to prevent a localized outbreak from becoming a national or even international nightmare.

The major drawback of much of the information currently available is that finding it frequently requires persistence and effort. Unfortunately, many agencies disseminating the data automatically assume that everyone is computer literate, familiar with the navigation of the Web, and has access to rapid downloads. All that may be true at the major medical centers, but many facilities have outdated computer systems, use antiquated and very slow modems, and, paradoxically enough, may have difficulties in accessing the Web because some system administrators still consider this a "business-unrelated" activity!

The difficulties in rapid access to the relevant medical information, particularly when such need is very urgent, became particularly evident while preparing a human patient simulator-based course on the management of bioterrorism-relevant diseases. During scenario development, we quickly realized that the needed data were sometimes difficult to find. Once found, they were often contained within bulky papers that required time to read. Frequently, the papers repeated each other uncritically, and often the data were simply too old and did not reflect the new thinking. Equally frustrating were the Web site crashes and "members only" access — a surprising discovery considering that data they contain may be vital to a healthcare provider suspecting the onset of a bioterrorism-like event.

Other Web sites required inordinate amounts of "fishing" before the relevant facts could be extracted. Frustrating as these discoveries were, and even if relatively short of time, our efforts to access the information were merely playacting rather than operating in the tense world of real medical activities following a bioterrorism attack. It is at this point we realized the need for a practical manual providing pertinent aspects of each disease relevant to bioterrorism: clinical features, required laboratory tests, recommended treatments, and outlines of precautionary measures.

The contents of the resulting manual will be trivial to a physician, nurse, scientist, or seasoned paramedic experienced in dealing with infectious diseases. Yet, a very large number of healthcare workers are strangers to the territory of the deadly contagious illnesses. Most lack familiarity with the presenting symptoms, and it is not surprising that what to a Puerto Rican physician is unmistakably dengue fever will appear as a benign flu to a physician in Michigan or North Dakota. Even more confusing, during their initial stages the majority of diseases relevant to bioterrorism are associated with highly nonspecific symptoms, often resembling those seen during a bad season of colds and influenzas. Only a keen observer will detect anomalies in presentation or the sheer frequency of identical cases and raise an alarm. Today, a high index of suspicion is a vital tool in outbreak prevention. How critical this attitude can be is exemplified by Dr. Larry Bush and his colleagues in Florida, without whom the consequences of mail dissemination of anthrax spores could have been significantly worse.

The present manual is not an exhaustive source of knowledge about any of the described diseases. It is a compilation of relevant information that does not offer anything that cannot be found in the electronic jungle of URL addresses. The purpose was to extract this information, put it together in a manner that would prove useful even in moments of the greatest stress, and create a book suitable for true field use. A book providing enough data to start a meaningful approach to patients that would in turn buy the time to locate experts and implement a winning strategy. An exhaustive list of Web-based resources is provided at the end of the manual, allowing the treatment provider to go to the sources and refine the treatment further.

The manual also contains sections on a number of techniques that may become useful. A brief refresher on simple microscope stain techniques can be quite handy in situations in which a "quick and dirty" approach may offer an extraordinarily useful hint. Moreover, it must not be forgotten that the environment of bioterrorism-related mass casualties may stretch the standard resources to the maximum. Hence, the ability to perform competently some of the basic lab procedures may be of sudden significance.

In summary, the manual is an introduction to the most essential operational aspects in the environment of a bioterrorist threat. It is aimed at nonspecialist medical personnel at all levels, i.e., physicians, nurses, paramedics, first responders, and all other participants within the classical EMS system. The goal was to provide them with a resource that can be thrown into a medical bag and kept there, hopefully forever unused but, if needed, a resource that can be rapidly opened to a relevant page providing the essential information to start the treatment, and maintain it until the expert assistance becomes available.

The manual would not exist without the efforts of medical scientists, physicians, and authors whose work was essential in preparing the present compilation. My colleagues at MedSMART whose forbearance, help, and willingness to assume many of my duties allowed me to concentrate on writing must also be acknowledged. Madeleine Leigh spent countless hours making the text both readable and easy to use, and I am grateful for her editorial assistance. My special gratitude goes to two women of almost legendary stubbornness and iron will: Mara J. and my mother. Mara J., a very senior member of the "healing professions," offered professional fellowship, trust, and support, all of which were sources of unending encouragement. However, it is her love that, ultimately, provided and continues to provide the most significant factor. My mother — a highly decorated nurse and surgeon in the Polish Underground during the Second World War, a poet, and a well-known actress — with her experiences, wisdom, and devotion to others always served as an example that influenced many of my professional decisions. Without discussions with her, this manual would never have seen the light of day.

AUTHOR

Dag K.J.E. von Lubitz, Ph.D., M.D. (Sc.) is chairman and chief scientist at MedSMART (Medical Simulation, Modeling, Advanced Research, and Training), Inc.

Dr. von Lubitz is a graduate of the University of Copenhagen and subsequently served as a fellow at the Department of Neuropathology, Royal Hospital, Copenhagen. In the U.S., he became a visiting associate in neuropathology at the National Institute of Neurological Disorders and Stroke (NINDS), at the National Institutes of Health (NIH), and a guest investigator in the Department of Neurobiology at the Uniformed Services University of Health Sciences (USUHS). After departure from NIH, Dr. von Lubitz served as a senior investigator and visiting associate professor with the ONR program at Hahnemann University, Philadelphia. He returned to the National Institute of Diabetes and Digestive and Kidney Disorders at NIH in 1990 as an associate scientist and visiting professor.

In 1997, Dr. von Lubitz joined the University of Michigan, serving as an assistant professor of surgery and emergency medicine, and director of the Emergency Medicine Research Laboratories. While at the university, he created the Medical Readiness Training (MRT) Laboratory and introduced the new concept of a "medical flight simulator" combining immersive virtual reality with high-fidelity patient simulation. In 2001, von Lubitz founded and became the chairman of the board and chief scientist of MedSMART, Inc. — the first organization in the U.S. devoted to research and medical training based on distributed simulation. Together with his colleagues at MedSMART, von Lubitz established the principles of global range interactive distance training based on remote access to the sophisticated training center in Ann Arbor, Michigan, using advanced telepresence and visualization techniques. A scientist with over 200 publications, von Lubitz is an internationally recognized keynote speaker, lecturer, and the recipient of U.S. and international research scholarships (Fellow,

Foundation for the Advancement of Science; Special Senior Fellow, Cystic Fibrosis Foundation; and Fellow, Royal Danish Medical Research Council Award). He also serves as a medical grant reviewer for several states of the European Community, and is an active member of several professional medical and technology societies in the U.S. and abroad. In 2000, von Lubitz became one of the laureates of the 2000 Smithsonian Computerworld Prize, and in 2002 he received two prestigious international awards — the Laval Virtuel Prize in Medicine and the City of Laval Prize for International Achievement in Advanced Technology. Von Lubitz is the author of the first simulation-based distributed training program for first responders offered in collaboration with Central Michigan University. He also devised the first training program on medical management of bioterrorism victims that is solely based on simulation and the principles of advanced distributed learning.

GLOSSARY OF MEDICAL TERMS

Adenopathy Swelling or enlargement of lymph nodes

Afebrile Without fever; having normal body temperature

Agglutination (test) Process in which suspended bacteria clump into larger aggregates

Alar Related to wings (alae) of structures such as the nose, sacrum, etc.

Anemia Condition in which the number of red blood cells in a given volume of blood is less than normal

Anorexia Diminished appetite or aversion to food

Antecubital In front of the elbow

Anuria Absence of urine formation

Aphasia Impairment or absence of speech or ability to communicate by means of writing or signs

ARDS Adult Respiratory Distress Syndrome

Arthralgia Severe joint pain

Arthrocentesis Aspiration of joint fluid through a puncture needle.

Ascites Accumulation of serous fluid in the peritoneal cavity

Ataxia Inability to coordinate movement

Axillar Related to the area of the armpit

Bacteremia Presence of viable bacteria in the blood

bid Twice a day

Bradycardia Slowness of heartbeat (by convention, less than 60 beats per minute)

Bubo Inflammatory swelling in a lymph node, typically in the groin.

CBC Complete blood count

Clubbing Thickening or widening of the distal segment of fingers and toes; the nails are abnormally curved and shiny

Consolidation Dense, firm mass in the lung

CT (scan) Computed tomography scan

CXR Chest x-ray

Cyanosis Dark or bluish discoloration of the skin or mucosa caused by inadequate oxygenation of blood

Cytotoxin Substance that prevents cell function or destroys cells.

Diaphoresis Perspiration

DIC Disseminated Intravascular Coagulation

Diplopia Double vision

Diuresis Production of urine; typically denotes abnormally large amounts

Dysarthria Disturbance of speech or language due to emotional stress, spasticity of muscles, or brain injury

Dyspepsia Impairment of gastric function; upset stomach

Dysphagia Difficulty in swallowing

Dysphonia Altered voice production

Dyspnea Shortness of breath, difficulty in breathing

Ecchymosis Purplish patch extending more than 3 mm across the skin caused by leakage of blood from blood vessels into the skin

ELISA Enzyme-Linked Immunosorbent Assay

Endocarditis Inflammation of the endocardium

Endotoxemia Presence of endotoxins (bacterial toxins that are not freely released into the surrounding medium) in the blood

Endotracheal Within the trachea

Epididymitis Inflammation of the epididymis (structure involved in transport, storage, and maturation of spermatozoa)

Epistaxis Profuse bleeding from the nose

Epitrochlear Related to the medial epicondyle (a projection near the articulating surface) of the humerus

Erythema Redness of skin caused by capillary dilatation

Erythroderma Intense, widespread reddening of skin due to dilatation of blood vessels

Eschar Thick, coagulated crust seen at the site of a burn or an anthrax-related skin lesion

Exudative pharyngitis Inflammation of pharyngeal muscosa and underlying structures associated with oozing of fluids (exudates) and formation of encrustations

Flaccid Relaxed, flabby

Fulminant Occurring very suddenly and with great intensity or severity.

g Gram (weight)

Gastroenteritis Inflammation of the mucous membranes of the stomach and intestine

Granulomatous Having characteristics of granuloma (a nodular lesion, typically small, firm, persistent, containing compactly associated mononuclear phagocytes)

Hematemesis Vomiting of blood

Hematogenous Anything produced or derived from blood or transported by blood

Hematuria Presence of blood in urine

Hemoptysis Spitting of blood derived from lungs or bronchial tubes

Hepatomegaly Enlargement of liver

Hypercapnia Abnormally increased tension of carbon dioxide in blood

Hyperesthesia Abnormal sensitivity to touch, pain

Hypotonia Reduced tone in any anatomical part (e.g., arteries, muscles)

IgG Immunoglobulin G

IgM Immunoglobulin M

Ileus Mechanical obstruction of the bowel; may be accompanied by severe pain, abdominal distention, absence of stool, fever, dehydration

IM Intramuscular injection

Induration Process of becoming extremely hard; presence of such characteristics in tissue

IV Intravenous injection

Lacrimation Secretion of tears

Laryngitis Inflammation of the larynx

Left shift Markedly increased number of immature cells in circulating blood

Leukocytic pleocytosis Increased number of leukocytes (more than 10,000 per cubic millimeter of blood) seen in acute infections and other pathological states

Leukocytosis See **leukocytic pleocytosis**

Leukopenia Reduced number of leukocytes (by convention, fewer than 4000 to 5000 per cubic millimeter) in circulating blood

Lymphadenopathy Disease process affecting lymph nodes

Lymphopenia Reduction in number of leukocytes in circulating blood

Macula Small, discolored spot (patch) on the skin that is neither depressed nor elevated above skin surface; plural is **maculae**

Maculopapule Lesion with a flat base that surrounds a papule

mg Milligram **(weight)**

Miliary nodule Nodule having the size of a millet seed (approximately 2 mm)

MR Magnetic resonance

Mucopurulent Exudate containing mostly pus, with an admixture of conspicuous amounts of mucous material

Multilobar Having several lobes

Myalgia Muscular pain

Mycoplasmal Pertaining to a genus of aerobic to facultative anaerobic Gram-negative bacteria (family Mycoplasmataceae)

Mydriasis Dilatation of the pupil

Myopathy Disease of muscular tissue; typically denotes a disorder of the skeletal musculature

Nephritis Inflammation of the kidneys

Neuropathy Disease involving cranial nerves or the peripheral or autonomous nervous system

Nosocomial Relating to a hospital; a new disorder such as an infection acquired during a stay at a hospital

Nuchal Relating to the nape of the neck

Ophthalmoplegia Paralysis of one or more ocular muscles

Oropharyngeal Related to the mouth and pharynx

ORS Oral Rehydration Solution

Osteomyelitis Inflammation of bone marrow and surrounding bone

Papula Small, circumscribed, solid elevation of the skin; plural is **papulae**

Parenteral Introduction of substances by other routes than the gastrointestinal tract, e.g., IV or IM injection

PCR Polymerase Chain Reaction

Petechiae Pinpoint- to pinhead-sized hemorrhagic spots in the skin that cannot be blanched by applied pressure

Pharyngitis Inflammation of the pharynx

Photophobia Aversion to light

Pleocytosis Presence of more cells than normal as in leukocytosis or lymphocytosis

Pleomorphic Occurring in more than one morphologic form

Pleuritic Pertaining to pleurisy (inflammation of the pleura)

Pneumonitis Inflammation of the lungs (pneumonia)

PO By mouth (per os)

Polyarthritic Simultaneous inflammation of several joints

Polyuria Excessive excretion of urine accompanied by very frequent urination

Prodrome Group of early symptoms of a disease that offer early warning of its forthcoming full development

Prostration Exhaustion; pronounced loss of strength

Proteinuria Urine protein in concentration higher than 0.3 g in a 24-hour collection period or greater than 1g/l in two or more random urine collections separated by at least 6 hours

Pruritus Itching

Ptosis Drooping of the eyelids

Purpura Condition characterized by hemorrhage into the skin; appearance varies depending on type of purpura, acuteness of onset, and duration of lesions

Pustula Small, circumscribed elevation on the skin with purulent contents; plural is **pustulae**

qd Each day

qid Four times a day

Retinitis Inflammation of retina

Retrosternal Posterior to (behind) the sternum

Rhinitis Inflammation of the mucous membranes of the nose

Rhinorrhea Discharge from the mucous membranes of the nose

Rigor Stiffness, rigidity

Sacroiliitis Inflammation of the sacroiliac joint

Splenitis Inflammation of the spleen

Splenomegaly Enlargement of the spleen

Stridor High-pitched respiratory sound indicating obstruction of the trachea or larynx

SC subcutaneous injection

Suppurative Pus-forming

Tachypnea Rapid breathing

Thrombocytopenia Abnormally low number of platelets in the circulating blood

tid Three times daily

Titer Standard of strength of a volumetric test solution; assay value of an unknown measure using volumetric testing

Tonsillar Relating to tonsils, in particular to the palatine tonsil

Vasculitis Inflammation of a blood vessel or lymphatic vessel

Vector In the context of this manual, an invertebrate animal (e.g., a tick or mosquito) that transmits an infectious pathogen among vertebrates

Vaccinia Infection, typically local and limited to the site of inoculation with *Vaccinia* (cowpox) to confer immunity to smallpox (Variola)

VIG Vaccinia immune globulin

Viremia Presence of a virus in the bloodstream

WBC White blood count

Zoonotic Relating to zoonosis; infection shared by humans and animals, the latter being its usual host; infection acquired by humans from animals

1

BRIEF OVERVIEW OF BIOLOGICAL WARFARE AND BIOTERRORISM

TERRORISM AS A THREAT

The principal goal of all terrorists is to undermine the existing structure of society so that it will be forced to accept their demands in order to avoid further destruction. Contrary to popular belief, acts of terrorism, particularly international terrorism, need not involve mass casualties similar to those resulting from wars between nations. Instead, terrorism bases its actions on swift, unpredictable assaults that force a target nation into a state of never-ending vigilance and redirection of its resources into sustained and costly counterterrorism measures that ultimately lead to prolonged economical and political turmoil.

Destabilization of the national fabric of life will eventually lead to the introduction of countermeasures that place further burdens on the population may cause internal strife, and induce racial and ethnic tensions, that will continue the process of destabilization. The goal of continual and targeted terrorism is to induce sufficient uncertainty to cause public and political pressure on the governing bodies to "open a dialogue" with the terrorists. Terrorist goals will thus acquire legitimacy by becoming "social grievances" that can be addressed only at the level of a national government or an international organization such as the United Nations (UN). Terror ultimately becomes sanctified as "democracy in action."

To attain legitimization of their goals, terrorist organizations need not resort to acts causing major catastrophic events involving hundreds of thousands of casualties resulting from, for example, the explosion of a nuclear device. On the scale of catastrophic events such as earthquakes or tropical cyclones, the events of September 11, 2001 constituted a series of relatively minor incidents. On the other hand, their gruesome nature — the fact that they represented the basest form of a terrorist act — sent a chilling message to the United States and the rest of the world. The subsequent release of anthrax spores through the mail system amplified the level of anxiety. Society has been forced to take actions that, even a very short time ago, would have been considered absurd. Moreover, counterterrorism measures have necessitated expenditure of billions of dollars that a free society could have spent on better causes in service of its citizens.

Had the September attacks been directed at a weaker, less unified nation with fewer resources, that nation would have collapsed and entered negotiations with the terrorists. Instead, the swift and forceful political and military responses of the U.S. government produced, probably for the first time in modern history, an international atmosphere ready to eliminate terror as a form of political dispute.

Despite severe weakening of Al-Qaeda and similar organizations, the threat of terrorist action has not disappeared. The wars against the Taliban and against the oppressive regime of Saddam Hussein may have intensified the threats by adding fuel to the already highly inflammatory and combative anti-Western rhetoric of militant Islam. The combination of the terrorism sponsorship by such states as Syria and Iran, and easy access to advanced technologies allows terrorist groups to conduct global war against the West with highly sophisticated means of assault.

Among the tools available to international terrorists, biological agents are probably the most surreptitious and emotionally devastating. Manufacture of suitable pathogens at a scale relevant to bioterrorism (as opposed to warfare) is relatively easy and does not require ultrasophisticated facilities. Some bioterrorism agents are available on the clandestine international weapons market. Since the collapse of the Soviet Union, almost any weapon within its former arsenal can be purchased. Furthermore, transport of biological agents across borders is easy because no detection system is capable of alerting immigration and customs officials to the passage across check points of small quantities of well concealed biological materials. Environmental release of some pathogens is simple to accomplish and easily disguised. Finally, the medical effects of contamination manifest after a relatively long incubation period, allowing the perpetrators enough time to escape.

Many thousands of casualties may be produced by a bioterrorist attack, but even a very small number of victims such as those who developed anthrax in the U.S. can produce a devastating societal impact and long-lasting psychological effects. The next time influenza epidemic strikes, the vision of bioterrorism will loom and exert massive and unnecessary fiscal and logistic strain on healthcare resources.

BIOTERRORISM IN HISTORY

Biological warfare has its roots in antiquity, when the practical applications of using biologically active agents on the battlefield were recognized. One of the earliest descriptions of battlefield use of biological weapons arose from the sea battle between the forces of Hannibal and King Eumenes of Pergamum (184 B.C.). Sailors on Hannibal's ships tossed earthen pots filled with venomous snakes on board the Eumenean vessels. The resultant terror and confusion among the Eumeneans assured Hannibal's rapid victory.

Throughout the Middle Ages, the easiest and most effective form of biological assault was contamination of water supplies by tossing corpses and carcasses of animals into wells and rivers supplying besieged cities. Siege warfare led to a new form of attack where rapid surrender was assured by catapulting plague-ridden bodies into besieged towns. The practice continued well into the 18th century. More gruesome examples of germ warfare evolved during the conquest of the Americas; smallpox was the primary offensive agent. Pizarro used variola-contaminated clothing to spread smallpox among South American Indians in the 15th century. The English used the same method and distributed smallpox-contaminated blankets to North American Indians during the wars conducted from 1754 through 1767. The resulting epidemic decimated tribes in the Ohio region. One of the lesser known facts about biological warfare is the introduction of mandatory smallpox vaccination by George Washington during the Revolutionary War.

The First World War gained the dubious honor of providing the stage for the introduction of chemical warfare. Unproven accusations that the Germans used anthrax and glanders as weapons against the U.S., and attempted to spread plague and cholera in Italy, Russia, and Romania, were rife at that time. The German military was also alleged to have dropped plague-contaminated chocolate and toys from airplanes in attempts to spread the disease among children. Subsequently, the League of Nations absolved the German forces of conducting germ warfare. However, the horrifying casualties resulting from the use of toxic gases on the battlefield led to the Geneva Protocol of 1925 prohibiting implementation of chemical and bacteriological agents in war. The protocol was signed by 108 nations. Libya and Iraq, future proponents of the use of chemical and biological weapons, were among the signatories. Late in the 20th century, Iraq employed chemical warfare agents in a war with Iran and against its own Kurdish population.

Although the Germans experimented with infectious diseases in warfare during the second World War (using Russian prisoners of war as guinea pigs), they were not charged with such offenses during the subsequent war crime trials. The Japanese, on the other hand, conducted extensive experimentation and actively participated in germ warfare against Chinese and Russian civilians and military units as early as 1939. Soon after the commencement of hostilities involving Japan, the U.S., and Great Britain, Unit 731 of the Japanese Imperial Army embarked on a series of very extensive experiments on Chinese and Mongolian civilians and prisoners of war. American, Australian, British, and Russian prisoners of war were also used to test the effects of various bacteriological agents. The "effectiveness" of these experiments was assured by the construction of special facilities in Manchuria, China, and Singapore. During post-war trials, the commanding officer of Unit 731 testified that each year up to 600 war prisoners were killed during the tests. On the Allied side, British trials of small munitions containing anthrax bacteria caused heavy and persistent contamination on Gruinard Island. The contamination prevented habitation on the island for several years after the war.

Numerous allegations of the use of bacteriological warfare agents by the Western Powers, particularly the U.S., ensued during and after the Korean War. However, declassified documents obtained from both sides indicate beyond a doubt that the allegations were nothing but propaganda spread by the Eastern Bloc. In 1970, South Korea accused North Korea of preparing biological attacks. The charges, based on North Korea's large purchase of several biological agents, were ultimately abandoned, but the rumors about using such agents in wars in Southeast Asia persist. "Yellow rain," a weaponized form of trichothecene mycotoxin purportedly used by North Vietnamese forces in Laos, remains controversial. On the other hand, the use of antipersonnel traps containing sharpened, feces-covered sticks is a well documented form of biological warfare used by the Viet Cong.

A major step in the control of germ warfare was the signing of the 1972 Convention on the Prohibition of the Development, Production, and Stockpiling of Bacteriological (Biological) and Toxin Weapons and Their Destruction, signed by 103 nations. The agreement became effective in March 1975, but contained a major loophole: the convention allowed defensive research to continue providing a convenient platform for the continuation of work on biological warfare agents and methods of their dissemination. The Soviet Union used this opportunity extensively and created a number of research facilities. The vast nature of the Soviet program came to the attention of the U.S. after an explosion at a research institute in Sverdlovsk that caused several deaths from inhalation of anthrax spores, and led to virtually total isolation of the region by the Soviet armed forces. Soviet authorities denied accidental release of anthrax spores into the atmosphere and claimed the cause was accidental contamination of meat. The truth emerged in 1992, when Boris Yeltsin confirmed long-held suspicions about atmospheric release.

Soviet intelligence services pioneered the operational terrorist use of biological agents by constructing ingenious umbrella-like explosive devices capable of inserting biotoxin-contaminated pellets into human targets. This close-range weapon was used at least twice against prominent Bulgarian exiles in France. Unconfirmed reports indicate that a similar assassination was attempted in Virginia.

Operations Desert Shield and Desert Storm and events during the subsequent decade brought the attention of the world back to the issues of threats posed by biological weaponry. Although Iraq did not use its capacity during the conflicts, the threat revealed serious deficiencies in the preparedness of the U.S. military to wage war in the presence of a large-scale battlefield release of biological agent. After surrender of the Iraqi forces, the United Nations instituted an inspection program (UNSCOM) that revealed convincing evidence of a major effort by Iraq directed at manufacturing and stockpiling a wide range of bioweapons.

The nations of the Desert Storm Coalition (particularly the U.S. and Great Britain) attempted to interrupt the Iraqi program of biowarfare through economic sanctions and direct military action, but many intelligence sources cited the continuing capacity of Iraq to wage war based on the use of biological agents via terrorism and in conventional military operations. Continuing failure by Saddam Hussein to eliminate Iraqi weapons of mass destruction and dismantle all relevant manufacturing and research programs led to a series of UN resolutions and renewed intensity of international inspection. Despite intense international pressure to accept UN resolutions and disarm, the government of Iraq persisted in its deception and ultimately led to Operation Iraqi Freedom, a military invasion by U.S. and British armed forces supported by units provided by a coalition of over 35 countries. Although the regime of Saddam Hussein has been dislodged, intelligence sources indicate possible presence of weapons of mass destruction in several countries of the Middle East. Despite the recent war, it remains to be seen whether the region has been permanently freed from threats of war waged by means of chemical and biological weapons.

While Libya, Syria, and possibly Iran are among the prime suspects that harbor Islamic fundamentalist groups willing to use biological agents in their terrorist activities, other subversive organizations eager to employ similar tactics have been uncovered in the countries as unlikely as Japan and France. Members of the Aum Shinrikyo cult released sarin in the Tokyo subway in 1995 and also prepared large quantities of *Clostridium difficile* intended for terrorist use. In France, a considerable supply of botulinum toxin was discovered in the Parisian safe house of a radical Red Army Faction.

Anthrax dispersal represents the latest in the history of bioterrorism in the U.S. The first reported event occurred in 1984 when members of the Bhagwan Shree Rajneesh cult attempted to poison several people in Dalles, Oregon, in order to eliminate opposition and win local elections. While no fatalities occurred, this largely underreported incident clearly indicated the vulnerability of the U.S. to the determined actions of a well-organized terrorist group. Several incidents of bioterrorist threats followed during the intervening years. In most cases, threats were not converted into actions, but real dangers materialized as results of a few incidents. In 1989, the U.S. Food and Drug Administration was forced to conduct its largest safety investigation while searching for contaminated fresh fruit following a threat by a terrorist wishing to draw the nation's attention to the plights of Chilean agricultural workers. In 1995, a white supremacist was found to possess explosive devices intended to disperse plague-causing bacteria (*Yersinia pestis*). Also in 1995, members of a militia group were convicted for planning to use ricin toxin against U.S. marshals and the Internal Revenue Service. Several hoaxes also were reported and, as evidenced by the arrest of a federal worker in an Eastern Seaboard state, the criminal attitude persists in a small circle of attention seekers. The most unfortunate consequence of bioterrorism hoaxes is the major dissipation of national resources needed to contain real threats.

The September 11 attacks and the discovery of anthrax-containing letters sent to several media organizations and to the Senate brought international terrorism to U.S. territory. Until September 11, few people paid much attention to the dangers of terrorism despite vivid pictures of victims from France, Ireland, Israel, Germany, and Spain. Even before the direct attack, the U.S. had clear indications that the danger of terrorist attack was real. Studies have shown that a bioterrorist assault would threaten the very fabric of U.S. society. In 2000, a highly realistic simulation exercise was performed in Denver. It involved release of plague bacteria into the ventilation ducts of the Performing Arts Center. By the end of the exercise 4 days later, the simulated epidemic spread beyond control. The estimated death toll was 1000 to 2000 people and nearly 4000 cases of nonfatal infections were projected. More importantly, the exercise demonstrated a virtually complete collapse of the local healthcare system, the government, and massive strain on law enforcement authorities. The lack of adequate preparedness among pre- and in-hospital healthcare providers in dealing with a major infectious disease outbreak caused by a highly virulent and easily transmitted agent was equally disconcerting.

The sobering results that emerged from Denver and similar tests point to the essential nature of appropriate training at all levels of the healthcare system. Today, authorities have no doubt that effective training is paramount for rapid identification of the disease, immediate initiation of the appropriate treatment, and the introduction of relevant isolation and containment procedures, all of which are crucial ingredients in preventing a small outbreak from becoming a national catastrophe.

2

PATHOGENS POSING MAJOR THREATS

CLASS A AGENTS

Class A agents include bacteria, viruses, flaviviruses, and toxins. They pose the most dangerous threats because they:

- Are disseminated easily from person to person
- Cause high mortality
- Cause serious social disruption and/or panic
- Require special preparedness measures

Bacteria

- Smallpox (*Variola major*)
- Anthrax (*Bacillus anthracis*)
- Plague (*Yersinia pestis*)
- Botulism (*Clostridium botulinum*)
- Tularemia (*Francisella tularensis*)

Viruses

Filoviruses (Filoviridae)

- Ebola hemorrhagic fever
- Marburg hemorrhagic fever
- Arenaviruses (Arenaviridae*)*

- Lassa fever
- Junin and related viruses (Argentinian hemorrhagic fever, Bolivian hemorrhagic fever [Machupo], Brazilian hemorrhagic fever [Sabia], and Venezuelan hemorrhagic fever [Guanarito])

Flaviviruses (Flaviviridae)

- Dengue hemorrhagic fever
- Other hemorrhagic fevers endemic to India, Africa, Russia, and parts of South America

Toxins

- Botulinum
- Trichothecene (T2) mycotoxins

CLASS B AGENTS

Class B agents include bacteria, viruses, and toxins. They pose intermediate threats because they:

- Are disseminated with moderate ease
- Cause low to moderate mortality and morbidity
- Require enhancements of disease surveillance and preparedness

Bacteria

- Q fever (*Coxiella burnetti*)
- Brucellosis (*Brucella* sp.)
- Glanders, melioidosis (*Burkholderia mallei*)

A subset of class B bacterial agents may be used as food and water contaminants. These include:

- *Salmonella* sp.
- Shigella dysenteria
- *Escherichia coli* strain O 157:H7
- Cryptosporidium parvum

Viruses

Alphaviruses (Togaviride Family)

- Venezuelan equine encephalitis (VEE)
- Eastern equine encephalitis (EEE)
- Western equine encephalitis (WEE)
- Other alphaviruses with worldwide distribution

Toxins

- Ricin toxin from castor beans (*Ricinus communis*)
- Epsilon toxin from *Clostridium perfringens*
- *Staphylococcus* enterotoxin B (SEB)

CLASS C AGENTS

Class C agents pose low to moderate threats and include emerging pathogens that *can* be weaponized because of their ready availability or potential for high mortality and morbidity. Class C agents include bacteria and viruses:

- Multidrug-resistant tuberculosis
- Nipah virus
- Hantaviruses
- Tick-borne hemorrhagic fever viruses
- Tick-borne encephalitis viruses
- Yellow fever

3

MEDICAL DIAGNOSIS AND INITIAL TREATMENT

INTRODUCTION

As indicated earlier, the list of potential bioterrorism agents is extensive. While certain bacteria and viruses cited on the list are suitable for weaponization and their uses may have devastating consequences, their employment in a terrorist attack may be less likely in part due to the complexity of production and/or effective dispersal methods. Nonetheless, it must be remembered that some terrorist organizations have significant financial resources at their disposal that allow them access to sophisticated facilities capable of developing suitable contamination devices. Moreover, the support of such activities by foreign states cannot be excluded. Hence, it is mandatory that all healthcare personnel become aware of the essential clinical aspects of possible, even if unlikely, infections.

The following descriptions of the clinical manifestations of diseases that can serve as bioterrorism tools are of necessity brief and provide essential information only. Readers who wish to acquire deeper knowledge of those issues are referred to Chapter 8 (Resources).

For the sake of clarity and ease of reference, the descriptions of individual agents will be divided into following sections:

- Signs and symptoms
- Clinical features
- Differential diagnosis (symptoms are cited alphabetically rather than systemically)
- Laboratory tests including imaging and other relevant diagnostic techniques

- Treatment (adult doses are shown; pediatric doses are covered in Chapter 4)
- Prophylaxis (if any)
- Precautionary measures

For the sake of rapid accessibility, much information appears in bulleted lists. **Bold face** type is used for important points that may assist in rapid recognition of a disease, its treatment, or other salient aspects of management. **CAPITALIZED BOLD FACE** type is used for information that is critical or relates to the health of the managing personnel.

GENERAL ASPECTS OF MEDICAL MANAGEMENT

Several factors make biological terrorism a particularly effective form of assault. The development of appropriate preparedness measures requires recognition of the fact that biological assault offers significant advantages to the terrorist compared to other forms of terrorist activity, for example:

1. The availability of a wide range of contagious diseases
2. Nonspecific symptoms that complicate diagnosis
3. Diagnostic uncertainties increased by endemic factors
4. Relatively short incubation periods that allow spread of disease
5. Inadequacy and labor intensity of detection systems
6. Inadequate training in pathogen recognition on the part of medical and other personnel
7. General lack of familiarity with medical operations in a biocontaminated environment
8. Limited range of self-treatment possibilities
9. Potential for mass casualties
10. Large numbers of long-term patients that will stress healthcare systems
11. Possible hoax and copycat activities that will further tax government and healthcare resources

It is imperative that all parties involved in responding to bioterrorism understand the characteristic aspects of infection caused by individual pathogens, pathologies that may accompany infections, and modes of transmission, diagnostics, and treatment. At the first indication of the probability of exposure to biological warfare agents, healthcare providers must consider vigorous implementation of several procedures dealing with patients:

reduced urinary output
renal insufficiency
respiratory failure
retinitis
rhinitis
rhinorrhea
rice water stool
rigors
salivation
seizures
sepsis without bubo formation
shock
skin, burning pain
skin lesions, centrifugal distribution
skin lesions, synchronous development
sneezing
somnolence
spasmodic muscle on tapping
splenomegaly
stiff neck
stridor
sudden progression/worsening
substernal discomfort
sunken eyes
sweats
swollen neck
symmetric neurological symptomatology
tachycardia
tachypnea
thirst
tingling lips, tongue, fingertips
tremor
urinary retention
vertebral osteomyelitis
vesicles
vomiting
weakness
weight loss

Differential Diagnoses

abdominal aneurysm
acute adenitis
anthrax
aortic dissection
ARDS
blistering warfare agents
bowel obstruction
brain abscess
bronchitis
brucellosis
carbamate
catscratch disease
cellulitis
cholecystitis
cholera
ciguatera toxin
CNS trauma

FIRST LOOK

Many bioterrorism-related diseases may initially appear as common and benign problems

Common Disorder	Bioterrorism Event
INFLUENZA	Inhalational anthrax
	Pneumonic plague
	Tularemia
	Viral Hemorrhagic Fever (VHF)
VIRAL GASTROENTERITIS	Gastrointestinal anthrax
	Botulism
	Viral Hemorrhagic Fever (VHF)
VARICELLA	Smallpox

LOOK FOR

No upper respiratory tract syndrome	INHALATIONAL ANTHRAX
Widened mediastinum on CXR	
Prosis, diplopia, dysphagia, dysphonia	BOTULISM
Symmetric, descending weakness	
Hemoptysis	PNEUMONIC PLAGUE
Synchrony in lesion progression:	SMALLPOX
macules → papules → vesicles → pustules	
Centrifugal distribution of lesions (higher density on the extremities than torso)	
Petechiae below blood pressure cuff	VIRAL HEMORRHAGIC FEVER (VHF)

Overview of the symptoms characterizing diseases relevant to bioterrorism. Not all symptoms may be seen upon presentation, especially as some are characteristic of the early stages of illness, while others appear later. The chart clearly indicates that many of the diseases may be easily misdiagnosed as an ill-defined febrile syndrome. Only the subsequent progress of the infection will reveal its characteristic landmarks. It is therefore essential that during the periods of heightened terrorism alerts, all healthcare personnel are particularly vigilant to any atypical presentation of otherwise common diseases.

The list of diseases that should be considered as a part of differential diagnosis is provided under the symptoms chart.

Symptom

Symptom	Ant 18	Bruc 22	Cho 26	Cla 30	Plag 35	Plag 35	Plag 36	Q F 39	Tula 43	Equ 48	Hem 55	Sma 63	Bot 68	Ric 75	SEB 80	Sax 84	T2 88
abdominal cramps		X	X		X						X				X		X
abdominal pain		X		X	X				X								
abscesses, arms and legs				X													
abscesses, internal organs		H[b]		X													
acidosis			X														
acral cyanosis							X							X			
acute pulmonary edema/injury																	X
adenopathy, cervical			X						X								
adenopathy, systemic					X				X		X			X			
airway necrosis																	
altered mental state																	
anemia	X																
anorexia								X			X						
aphasia		X												X		X	X
arthralgia																	
asymptomatic									X								X
ataxia																	
back pain		X			X		X					X					X
black/tarry stools						X	X										X
blistering																	
blurred vision				X													
bronchopneumonia					X	X[a]											X
bubos																	
burning skin pain																	
chest discomfort	X																
chest pain, pleuritic									X					X			
chest tightness																	
chest wall edema																	
chills		X			X	X	X	X	X	X					X		
circulatory collapse						X		X									
clubbing																	
confusion										X			X	X			
conjunctival infection								X		X	X						
congestive heart failure					X	X	X	X	X								
constipation													X				
cough	X	X			X	X	X	X	X					X	X		X
cough, bloody/purulent						X											
cranial nerve palsies											X		X				
cyanosis					X	X								X			
delirium												X					
dehydration			X														
dementia																	
depression		X															
diaphoresis	X		X	X							X	X	X		X		X
diarrhea			X														
diarrhea (fulminant)			X														
diarrhea, bloody													X				
diplopia											X		X				
dizziness																	
drowsiness			X														
dry mouth						X							X				
dyspnea													X	X	X		X
dysarthria												X					
dyspepsia		X															
dysphagia													X				
dysphonia													X				
ecchymosis							X										
edema, peripheral		X						X			X				X		X
endocarditis																	

Symptom

Symptom	ANT 18	BRU 22	CHO 26	GLA 30	PLB 35	PLP 35	PLS 36	Q 39	TUL 43	EQ 48	HEM 55	SM 63	BOT 68	RIC 75	SEB 80	SAX 84	T2 88
necrosis	X																
necrosis, liver														X			
neurological aspects		X											X				
nonproductive cough	X									X							
nuchal rigidity										X							
numbness																X	
ophthalmoplegia													X				
osteomyelitis		X		X													
papulae					X												
papulae=vesicle=black eschar	X																
paralysis								X		X							
percussive dullness																	
petechiae							X				X						
pharyngitis									X		X						
pharyngitis, ulcerative																	X
photophobia				X						X							
pleuritic chest pain		X		X				X			X						
pleural effusions						X											
pneumonia, hemorrhagic						X											
positive tourniquet test																	
prostration									X		X	X		X	X		X
pruritus																	
ptosis													X				X
pulmonary edema														X	X		
pustules												X					
rash				X							X						X

Increased vigilance is essential for early detection of a pathogen. Speed increases the chances of saving patients' lives. Unfortunately, in many cases, prodromal (early phase) symptoms are nonspecific, making proper diagnosis difficult.

Increased levels of self-protection are essential to prevent accidental exposure to pathogens. A properly donned surgical mask offers a degree (albeit minimal in some cases) of such protection; the same is true for wearing gloves, covering exposed skin, buttoning lab coats, etc. Immunization and antibiotic prophylaxis may be implemented if the type of the pathogen can be anticipated with reasonable certainty.

Patients must be immediately assessed for airway, breathing, and circulatory adequacy. This should be followed by specific questioning concerning past medical history, present complaints, occupational history, exposure to vectors of disease (e.g., animals, insects, people with similar problems), immunization history, and recent food and liquid intake (where, what type). Physical examination should focus on the pulmonary and neuromuscular systems and unusual dermatologic and vascular features.

Although suspicion of exposure to a pathogen may be confirmed during physical examination, decontamination may not be necessary unless specific indicators of direct contamination are found (the presence of powders, liquid droplets, or stains, proximity to the site of pathogen release, etc.). In such cases, thoroughly showering the patient with copious quantities of soap and water may be sufficient. Sodium hypochlorite in 0.5% solution is recommended for decontamination of clothing but should be avoided as a means of skin decontamination. Contaminated clothing must be placed in tightly closed, double plastic trash disposal bags or containers and removed by assisting personnel (who should be dressed in appropriate skin and respiratory protective gear). Removal must be conducted in a manner that prevents secondary exposure of uncontaminated patients.

Definitive diagnosis must be performed on the basis of clinical, epidemiological, and laboratory findings. Access to essential laboratory tests in field or prehospital environment may be minimal or nonexistent. Hence, every attempt must be made to collect diagnostic nasal/throat swabs, blood, urine, and sputum samples and, if relevant, environmental swabs and samples. Particular attention must be paid to proper identification of the sampled materials.

In austere environments or when time is of the essence, syndromic diagnosis may be the only form of early determination of a pathogen. It must be kept in mind, however, that, with few exceptions, biological agents present with delays ranging from hours to days. Even then, the range of clinical syndromes may be limited. The difficulty in determining the nature of the biological agent is amplified by the following facts:

1. Plague, tularemia, and staphyloccal enterotoxin B (SEB) may present as pneumonia.
2. Upon presentation of botulism and Venezuelan equine encephalomyelitis (VEE), peripheral and central neuromuscular findings (respectively) may be present.
3. Brucellosis, Q fever, and VEE may present as undifferentiated febrile sdyndromes.
4. Anthrax, plague, tularemia, and smallpox have undifferentiated febrile prodromes.

Prompt treatment is essential in all cases. In resource-austere environments or when dealing with mass casualties, empirical treatment (i.e., immediate antibiotic treatment) may be the only approach available. Doxycycline (100 mg/PO/bid or as IV load at 200 mg followed by 100 mg IV q 12 hours) has been found effective for treating anthrax, plague, tularemia, brucellosis, and Q fever. Tetracyclines may also be considered.

In summary, the empirical approach may be considered in patients presenting with respiratory difficulties associated with undifferentiated febrile illness. **Such a form of treatment serves the purpose of initial antibiotic support and DOES NOT substitute for definitive treatment following final determination of the bioagent involved**. The details of definitive treatments are provided in the sections dealing with individual diseases.

Environmental precautions must be observed under all circumstances. Standard precautionary measures are sufficient for anthrax, tularemia, brucellosis, Q fever, VEE, and toxin exposure. While these diseases are not known to be contagious, practitioners are not absolved from extra vigilance against accidental exposure to the pathogen through contact with contaminated samples, clothing, etc. Smallpox requires airborne contagion precautions. Droplet protective measures must be used in the environments of smallpox and plague, while contact and droplet precautions are required in the presence of certain viral hemorrhagic fevers (VHFs) such as Ebola or Marburg.

Authorities must be alerted as soon as the suspicion of a bioterrorism-related event exists. The sooner such an alert is initiated, the greater the chance of reducing casualties and containing the outbreak. Early alert allows more efficient tracking of individuals who may have been exposed to the biological agent and left the area. It also improves the efficiency of all prophylactic measures.

Epidemiological assessment is equally essential from the outset. In all interviews with patients, healthcare workers must attempt to determine the circumstances surrounding the disease, exposure to and the nature of food and liquid sources, contacts with animals and people, and the history of physical movements. All these facts provide critical information to enable rapid implementation of appropriate prophylactic measures and tracking the disease to its origin, and may also assist in identifying the perpetrators and preventing recurrences.

The list of relevant diseases presented in this chapter is by no means complete. It is merely indicative of the variety of plausible agents. Moreover, medical personnel must bear in mind the possibility that the bacterial and viral pathogens involved in an incident may have been genetically manipulated in order to increase their virulence and resistance to pharmaceuticals or enhance their resistance to the environment outside the host, or to common decontamination agents. **If the behavior of a biological agent in a clinical setting is different from that described in the standard literature, the behavior must be considered as possible evidence of bioterrorism and must be reported to the appropriate authorities (Centers for Disease Control, Federal Bureau of Investigation) as soon as the observation is made. The report must be accompanied by appropriate nasal and throat swab samples, blood, serum, and urine samples, and biopsy and autopsy tissue samples.**

Bacterial Diseases

ANTHRAX

This zoonotic disease (transmissible from animals to humans under normal conditions) is caused by *Bacillus anthracis,* a Gram-positive rod-shaped bacterium. The typical route of infection is via contact with infected animals (cattle, sheep, goats, horses) or contaminated animal products (hides, wool, hair, flesh, blood, or excreta). Under natural conditions, infection with anthrax manifests as a skin lesion. When used as a bioterrorist or warfare agent, anthrax is dispersed as an aerosol or as spore dust. Spores are stable and resistant to sunlight for relatively long periods. Sudden worsening and/or deaths of patients originally presenting with flu-like symptoms indicate possible anthrax infection and demand immediate precautionary measures.

Signs and Symptoms

General Symptoms

- **Incubation period** is usually 1 to 6 days but may be significantly longer
- **Onset** of fever, nonproductive cough, malaise, fatigue, and occasional chest discomfort is gradual and nonspecific
- **Occasionally after a brief period of apparent improvement** (a characteristic sign of anthrax), a sudden progression to severe respiratory distress with dyspnea, diaphoresis, stridor, cyanosis, and shock occurs
- **Death** typically occurs 24 to 36 hours after the onset of severe symptoms

Specific Features

Inhalational Anthrax

- Physical findings are nonspecific on presentation (see above) but may include pleural effusions, chest wall edema, and meningitis
- At a later stage, dramatically widened mediastinum can be noted on chest x-rays (**CHARACTERISTIC SIGN**)

- Pleural (hemorrhagic) effusions are frequent, no infiltrates; the disease may be associated with hemorrhagic meningitis (**CHARACTERISTIC SIGN**)

Cutaneous Anthrax

- Most frequently on hands and forearms of people working with infected animals; inoculation through skin lacerations, abrasions, or fly bites
- Begins as papulae transforming into a liquid-filled vesicle that rises and forms a black eschar (scab); *anthrax* means *coal* (color of the eschar) in Greek
- Bacilli from the vesicular lesion can be observed with Gram stain
- Local infection can become systemic and fatal

Oropharyngeal and Gastrointestinal Anthrax

- Caused by ingestion of undercooked infected meat
- Incubation period is 2 to 5 days
- When untreated, mortality may be 50%

Orophanryngeal Anthrax

- Severe sore throat
- Local oral or tonsillar ulcer (diagnostic landmark)
- Fever
- Cervical or submandibular lymphadenitis and edema (swollen neck)
- Dysphagia and respiratory distress may be present

Gastrointestinal Anthrax

- Extremely difficult to diagnose
- Nonspecific nausea, vomiting, fever; severe abdominal pain
- May present as acute abdomen associated with hematemesis, massive ascites, and diarrhea

Differential Diagnosis

- Abdominal aneurysms
- Aortic dissection
- Coccidioidomycosis
- Diphtheria

■ Gastroenteritis
■ Meningitis
■ Pleural effusions
■ Pneumonia (bacterial, mycoplasmic, or viral)
■ Subarachnoid hemorrhage
■ Superior vena cava syndrome

Laboratory Tests

■ Gram stain: bacteria appear as large, Gram-positive rods
■ Serology assists only in retrospective diagnosis
■ Cerebrospinal fluid: blood and leukocytosis in meningeal involvement
■ Chest x-ray: mediastinitis with pleural effusions (**CHARACTERISTIC SIGN,** late stages), absence of typical pneumonia findings
■ Technetium 99-labeled monoclonal antibody method suitable for the detection of the earliest stages of inhalational anthrax is in clinical trial at Walter Reed Army Hospital in Washington, DC; it promises detection in asymptomatic patients much earlier than possible by current laboratory and radiological techniques

Treatment

Immediate Treatment

■ **Ciprofloxacin** (400 mg IV q 12 hours) oral administration is ineffective
■ **Doxycycline** (200 mg IV load, followed by 100 mg IV q 12 hours) oral administration is ineffective
■ **Penicillin G** (8 to 12 million units IV divided q 4–6 hours) may be an alternative after establishing absence of sensitivity

Maintenance Treatment

■ Continue treatment for 4 weeks after symptoms resolve
■ Ciprofloxacin (750 mg PO bid) or doxycycline (100 mg PO q 12 hours)
■ Supportive therapy for shock, fluid volume deficit, and adequate airway may be required

Prophylaxis

- Immunization: vaccine available but not for general use
- Oral antibiotics for 8 weeks (ciprofloxacin 500 mg bid; doxycycline 100 mg bid; amoxicillin 500 mg PO q 8 hours continued for at least 4 weeks)
- Levofloxacin and ofloxacin are NOT recommended

Precautionary Measures

Prehospital Measures

- Field decontamination of patients and exposed personnel if possible
- Copious amounts of soap and water should be adequate. Do not use bleach solutions
- If environmental presence of anthrax bacilli or spores is suspected, add dermal protection, gloves, and respirator with HEPA filter or self-contained breathing apparatus
- Place contaminated clothing in sturdy (triple) plastic bags; secure bags with individual closures; decontaminate outside surfaces with 0.5% hypochlorite solution (1 part household bleach, 9 parts water)

Hospital Measures

- Standard precautions; barrier nursing
- Isolation is not necessary
- Secretion precautions are recommended
- Skin lesions may pose risk of infection

Inhalational anthrax is not contagious. Nonetheless, during initial contact, extra caution should be exercised due to the possible contamination from spores in patient clothing, etc. All instruments used in invasive procedures and autopsies must be thoroughly disinfected with 0.5% sodium hypochlorite (see Chapter 5). Note: Hypochlorite strength is substantially reduced in the presence of organic material. Disposables must be placed in sealable containers containing sporicide, sealed, and removed from the area in a manner that prevents accidental contamination of clean sections of the facility.

BRUCELLOSIS

Brucellosis is a zoonotic disease of domestic and wild animals caused by bacteria belonging to the *Brucella* genus. Four species of these Gram-negative bacteria cause disease in humans. In aerosol form, the bacteria are highly infectious. Only 10 to 100 organisms are sufficient to cause disease in humans. The disease has a low (5% of untreated cases) mortality rate, with deaths, typically due to endocarditis or meningitis. It may be incapacitating and even disabling. Frequently it becomes chronic and may relapse despite treatment.

Approximately 200 cases of brucellosis are reported each year in the U.S. Occupation-related infections are the most common causes of the disease in the U.S. In other countries, consumption of unpasteurized dairy products (cheese in particular) is the main reason for high incidence of brucellosis.

Human-to-human transmission has not been reported, but high infection rates through inhalation are reported among laboratory workers involved in culturing *Brucellae*. **Due to the highly infective potential of aerosol-dispersed *Brucellae* and symptoms that can be easily misdiagnosed as influenza, brucellosis represents a significant potential threat.**

Signs and Symptoms

- Variable incubation period (5 to 60 days)
- Onset may be abrupt
- Presents as nonspecific febrile illness easily mistaken for influenza
- Fever
- Headache
- Myalgia
- Arthralgia
- Back pain
- Sweats
- Chills
- Generalized weakness and malaise
- Nonproductive cough and pleuritic chest pain if respiratory infection is present
- GI complaints include dyspepsia (typical) and abdominal pain (typically associated with hepatic abscess)
- Right upper quadrant pain and jaundice indicate hepatic abscess
- Neuropsychiatric complaints include depression, headaches, and irritability

- Meningoencephalitis is possible in advanced cases along with neurological deficits, nuchal rigidity, seizures, and coma
- Dermal findings (ulcerations, petechiae, purpura, erythema nodosum) are present

Clinical Features

- High suspicion index necessary for firm diagnosis
- Cough and pleuritic pain in up to 25% of cases; pulmonary symptoms do NOT correlate with chest x-ray
- Lymphadenopathy in 10 to 20% of cases
- Splenomegaly in 20 to 30% of cases
- Lumbar pain and tenderness in 60% of cases
- Low to normal leukocyte counts
- Anemia and thrombocytopenia have been reported
- Persistent fever despite treatment of prolonged musculoskeletal complaints requires CT/MR imaging
- Prolonged musculoskeletal complaints require CT/MR imaging
- Vertebral osteomyelitis, intervertebral disc space infection, paravertebral abscess, and sacroiliac infection occur as complications; sacroiliac joints most typically involved; hips, knees, and ankles may be involved
- Endocarditis in late stages
- Weight loss in chronic cases (>3 to 6 months) may be present

Differential Diagnosis

- Brain abscess
- Bronchitis
- Endocarditis
- Epididymitis
- Gastroenteritis
- Lumbar disk disorders
- Meningitis
- Pneumonia (bacterial, mycoplasmic, or viral)
- Sacroiliitis
- Subarachnoid hemorrhage
- Tuberculosis
- Tularemia
- Typhus
- Urinary tract infection
- Vasculitis

Laboratory Tests

- Complete blood count (CBC)
- Blood and bone marrow cultures give yields sufficient for definitive identification
- Antibody testing (most reliable method)
- Agglutination test (titers of 1:160 indicate positive diagnosis)
- Enzyme-linked immunosorbent assay (ELISA)
- Urine analysis and culture; sterile pyuria
- Arthrocentesis (excluding septic arthritis)
- Chest x-ray (usually normal)
- Cranial CT scan if altered mental status or focal neurological deficits are apparent; brucella-induced leptomeningitis, subarachnoid hemorrhage, or cerebral abscess may be present

Treatment

Oral antibiotics: consult an infectious disease specialist for definitive regimen.

Regimens of Choice

- Doxycycline 200 mg/qd PO plus rifampin 600 mg/qd PO for 6 weeks
- Doxycycline 200 mg/qd PO (6 weeks) plus streptomycin 1 g/qd IM for 2 weeks

Alternative Regimens

Other regimens involving doxycycline and gentamicin, TMP/SMX (trimethoprimsulphamethoxazole) and gentamicin, and ofloxacin with rifampin given for 4 to 6 weeks have been less effective. Surgery may be used in exceptional cases (localized disease).

Prophylaxis

- No licensed human vaccine available (veterinarian forms used widely)
- Chemoprophylaxis not recommended

Precautionary Measures

Standard precautions should be exercised in patient contact since no direct transmission from person to person has been reported. **However, the infectious potency of *Brucellae* is very high. When recent exposure of a patient to aerosolized *Brucellae* is suspected in a biological warfare or terrorism setting, extra caution is required to prevent secondary contamination through inhalation of bacteria released from clothing, etc.**

Due to inhalation danger present during testing of laboratory cultures of *Brucellae*, all work with these bacteria MUST be conducted with strict adherence to Biosafety Level 3 (BSL-3) rules.

CHOLERA

This disease is caused by *Vibrio cholera*, a Gram-negative, slightly curved bacillus whose motility is provided by a single polar flagellum. *Vibrio* species, including *V. cholera* and many noncholera species that can produce disease in humans, are among the most common organisms in surface waters and can be found in both fresh and salt water habitats. Although large-scale epidemic outbreaks of cholera were reported in the 1990s in South and Central America and in Asia, the incidence of the disease in the U.S. is low and most cases are related to foreign travel. Humans acquire the disease through ingestion of water or food contaminated with the bacilli. The most likely use of cholera bacteria in the context of biological warfare or bioterrorism is by contaminating water or food supplies. Dissemination in aerosol form is unlikely.

Noncholera *Vibrio* infections have been reported in Alabama, Florida, Louisiana, and Texas. **Septicemia is caused by food ingestion (primarily uncooked or undercooked shellfish). *V. vulnificus* produces the highest mortality rate (39%) among all cases of infection with noncholera Vibrio species**. While a sudden increase in *Vibrio* infections among inland populations with limited access to salt water may be indicative of a potential bioterrorism-related event, the possibility of natural contamination (particularly during the warmer months) must be considered.

Signs and Symptoms

- Incubation period: a few hours to 5 days
- May present as mild or fulminant diarrhea with fluid loss of 5 to 10 l/day or more
- Stool volume >250 ml/kg/24 hours
- Fecal matter during early course
- "Rice water" appearance **(CHARACTERISTIC SIGN)**
- Abdominal cramps
- Vomiting during early and late courses
- Reduced urinary output
- If untreated, may result in circulatory collapse

Clinical Features (Severe Cases)

- Severe dehydration may develop within hours
- Severe diarrhea
- Dry mouth and thirst

- No tears, sunken eyes
- Absent or barely palpable pulse
- Hypotension
- Tachycardia
- Tachypnea
- Hypercapnia
- Hypothermia
- Hypoglycemia (lethal complication in children)
- Acidosis **(possibility of normal serum [K⁺] in children when first seen; hypokalemia may develop when acidosis is corrected)**
- Spasmodic muscle contractions when supplying nerves are tapped (Chvostek/Trusseau signs) often present

Differential Diagnosis

- Gastroenteritis
  - *Bacillus cereus*
  - *Clostridium perfringens*
  - *Escherichia coli*
  - *Staphylococcus aureus*
- Other *Vibrio* infections

Laboratory Tests

Stool Microscopy

- Gram stain negative
- Characteristic motility only in dark field phase contrast microscopy

Stool Culture

- Use TCBS (thiosulphate-citrate-bile-sucrose) medium; large, smooth, round, and yellow colonies
- Many media used to culture enteric bacteria do not support *V. cholera* growth

Serum

- Sodium 130 to 135 mmol/l
- Potassium often normal in acute phase

- Bicarbonate << 15 mmol/l; may be undetectable
- BUN elevated
- Creatinine elevated

Treatment

Suspected Cases (Before Definitive Diagnosis)

- Assess dehydration
- Rehydrate under frequent monitoring
- Maintain hydration and replace fluid loss until diarrhea stops
- Administer antibiotic: tetracycline (250 mg PO q 6 hours for 3 to 5 days); doxycycline (200 mg PO initially followed by 100 mg q 12 hours for 3 to 5 days); ciprofloxacin (30 mg/kg divided in two doses for 3 days)
- Feed

Severe Cases

- Start IV line immediately
- Ringer's lactate solution; if not available, use normal saline
- If patient cannot drink, give oral rehydration salt (ORS) solution
  - *Patient >1 year old: 30 ml/kg within 30 minutes, then 70 ml/kg in the next 2 hours*
  - *Patient <1 year old: 30 ml/kg within 30 minutes, then 70 ml/kg in the next 5 hours*
- Monitor frequently; after initial 30 ml/kg, pulse should be strong and blood pressure normal; if not, continue IV fluid
- Administer ORS solution (5 ml/kg) as soon as the patient can drink
- Reassess adults 3 hours after start of rehydration and infants 6 hours after start of rehydration
- If signs of dehydration persist, maintain hydration using standard guidelines

Prophylaxis

- Previously available parenteral vaccine has little efficacy and is not recommended during outbreaks
- Suspension of killed *V. cholera* provides approximately 50% protection lasting ≤6 months; initial two doses given at least 2 weeks apart followed by booster shot every 6 months
- Oral live vaccines are experimental and still being tested

Precautionary Measures

Strict barrier nursing is recommended. Cholera is not transmittable other than by ingestion of contaminated food or water. Its symptoms are easily recognizable especially in adult patients, where no other disease can produce similarly intense dehydration. However, it has been suggested that in the U.S. the lack of practical experience with cholera may result in the differential diagnosis of severe gastroenteritis.

GLANDERS AND MELIOIDOSIS

These are zoonotic diseases. Glanders is caused by *Burkholderia mallei* and meliodiosis is caused by *B. pseudomallei*. Both are Gram-negative and present a "safety-pin" appearance. Infection in animals and humans is caused by inhalation or contamination of injuries. *B. mallei* induces disease in horses, mules, and donkeys. The rare instances of human infection are typically reported in veterinarians, horse and donkey handlers, and slaughterhouse workers.

B. mallei is common in tropical and subtropical regions and endemic in Southeast Asia and Australia. Presentation in humans varies from subclinical to massive septicemia resulting in 90% mortality within 24 to 48 hours. Pathogens invade nasal, oral, and conjunctival mucous membranes, enter the lungs through inhalation, or penetrate through skin injuries. Following incubation, patients present with symptoms of acute pulmonary infection or acute fulminant and ultimately fatal sepsis. Combinations have been reported.

Melioidiosis may remain dormant following primary infection. Patients may exhibit the acute form several years later. Immunological compromise is often associated. High infection rates caused by aerosols from cultures have been observed in laboratory workers, and cases of person-to-person transmission have been reported.

Signs and Symptoms

- Incubation period: 1 to 14 days depending on dose and agent virulence
- Septicemia begins suddenly
- Commonly associated with the disease are fever, rigors, sweats, myalgia, pleuritic chest pain, granulomatous or necrotizing lesions, erythroderma, jaundice, photophobia, lacrimation, and diarrhea
- Physical examination may reveal fever, tachycardia, cervical adenopathy, and mild hepatomegaly or splenomegaly

Clinical Features

Pulmonary Form

- Follows inhalation or hematogenous spread
- May be revealed by chest x-ray
  - *Miliary nodules*
  - *Bilateral bronchopneumonia*
  - *Segmental or lobar pneumonia*

    – Consolidation
    – Cavitating lesions

Mucosal (Localized) Form

- Mucopurulent, blood-streaked discharge from nose
- Septal/turbinate nodules and ulcerations

Septicemia Stage

- Systemic invasion originating from pulmonary, mucosal, or cutaneous infection leads to papular/pustular rash that **may be mistaken for smallpox**
- Abscesses in internal organs (brain, liver, spleen)
- Rapidly developing septic shock
- High mortality

Chronic Form

- Cutaneous and intramuscular abscesses on arms and legs
- Enlargement and induration of regional lymph nodes and channels
- Possible osteomyelitis, meningitis, and cerebral abscesses
- Asymptomatic cases are known

Differential Diagnosis

- Anthrax
- Plague
- Pneumonia (bacterial, mycoplasmic, viral)
- Smallpox
- Melioidosis should be always considered a possibility in differential diagnosis of any febrile illness associated with multiple pustular or subcutaneous lesions, fulminant respiratory failure, chest x-ray reminiscent of tuberculosis, and without Gram-negative bacteria present on sputum smears

Laboratory Tests

- CBC: mild leukocytosis with left shift or leukopenia
- Gram stain of blood, sputum, urine, and skin lesions
- Small, Gram-negative bacilli

- Irregular staining in methylene blue
- Blood cultures usually negative
- Agglutination tests are difficult interpretation due to high background titers
- Complement fixation test in melioidiosis: fourfold increase in titer is considered positive; a single titer above 1:160 indicates active infection
- Complement fixation test in glanders: titer ≥1:20 considered positive

Treatment

Treatment varies depending on the type and severity of the disease.

Localized Form/Mild Toxicity

- Amoxicillin and clavunalate: 60 mg/kg/day PO divided tid
- Tetracycline: 40 mg/kg/day PO divided tid
- TMP/SMX: TMP 4 mg/kg/day; SMX 20 mg/kg/day, PO tid
- Combination of two regimens is recommended for the initial 30 days, then monotherapy with amoxicillin/clavunalate or TMP/SMX for the next 60 to 150 days

Severe Disease

- Parenteral ceftazidime 120 mg/kg/day divided tid plus TMP/SMX (8 mg/kg/day TMP and 40 mg/kg/day SMX) divided qid
- Parenteral treatment for 14 days followed by PO therapy for 6 months
- If plague cannot be ruled out when treatment is initiated, add streptomycin (30 mg/kg/day IM; must not exceed 2.0 g/day)
- Doxycycline, rifampin, and ciproflaxin have been used in animal and *in vitro* studies. No human data are available

Prophylaxis

- No vaccine available for human use
- Postexposure prophylaxis with TMX/SMX may be contemplated

Precautionary Measures

- **Barrier protection with secretion precautions. Extra care needed due to the highly infectious potencies of both pathogens and the possibility of person-to-person transmission.** Environmental protection with 0.5% hypochlorite solution
- Biosafety Level 3 containment required for laboratories working with these pathogens
- Unless infection is due to attack by an animal or is directly related to work (glanders) or travel (melioidosis), the possibility of bioterrorism-related exposure is very likely

PLAGUE

Throughout its association with the human race, pandemic eruptions of plague led to sweeping societal changes at a cost of almost 200 million lives. The disease has never been eradicated and is present throughout the western to central U.S., where the number of reported cases appears to increase steadily. In the U.S., over 50% of cases are men less than 20 years of age who were infected within a 1-mile radius of home. Infections typically occur between April and November, peaking in July. Epizootic cycles occur every 5 years. It is predicted that a new epizootic outbreak may occur any time and may produce increased levels of human infections.

Plague is a zoonotic disease of rodents (rat, mice, ground squirrels) caused by *Yersinia pestis* (fam. Enterobacteraceae). Fleas living on rodents spread the disease to humans. However, transmission may also take place via inhalation of aerosol or close contact with contaminated tissue or fluid. The characteristic bubonic form of human plague may progress to septicemic and/or pneumonic form.

Infection typically takes place through the transfer of the pathogen from (usually) rat flea (*Xenopsylla cheopis*) to the skin of the victim. The bacillus invades nearby lymphoid tissue, producing the characteristic bubo — an inflamed, necrotic, hemorrhagic, and intensely painful lymph node. Subsequent spread follows the lymphatic channels in the direction of the thoracic duct and subsequent invasion of vasculature. Bacteremia and septicemia follow, and practically every organ may be invaded. The three forms of plague are bubonic, pneumonic, and septicemic.

Signs and Symptoms

- Onset 2 to 10 days following exposure
- Fulminant, nonspecific symptoms:
  - *Fever*
  - *Chills*
  - *Myalgia*
  - *Sore throat*
  - *Headache*
  - *Weakness*
  - *Malaise*
  - *Shortness of breath*
  - *Cough, at times producing bloody sputum*
  - *Nausea and (at times) bloody vomiting*
  - *Constipation, diarrhea, black or tarry stools*
- Stiff neck upon meningial infiltration by bacillus

Clinical Features

A sudden increase in the number of patients presenting with severe, rapidly progressing pneumonia with hemoptysis suggests outbreak of plague. However, diagnosis may be extremely difficult in individual patients presenting without bubos, especially in nonendemic regions. Differential diagnosis may be complex. **Demonstration of Gram-negative bacilli in the sputum indicate *Y. pestis* infection — the only Gram-negative bacterium that causes fulminant pneumonia with bloody sputum**.

Bubonic Plague

- Presence of characteristic bubos (swollen, at times extremely painful lymph nodes typically less than 5 cm); bubos are most commonly seen at the site of femoral and inguinal nodes (60%), and less frequently in the cervical and epitrochlear region
- Diffuse abdominal pain
- Liver and spleen may be tender and palpable
- Skin lesions in at least 25% of patients: pustules, vesicles, papulae containing leukocytes and bacteria, eschars

All are in the lymphatic drainage area of the affected node. Lesions are discovered frequently during autopsies.

Pneumonic Plague

- Acute and fulminant onset
- Presence of rare cervical bubos
- Diffuse crackles and areas of percussive dullness
- Cough with bloody, occasionally purulent, sputum
- Dyspnea, stridor, cyanosis
- Multilobar hemorrhagic and necrotizing pneumonia
- Gastrointestinal symptoms listed in the preceding section
- Meningitis and possible mental status changes (mild confusion to coma)
- Respiratory failure
- Circulatory collapse

Septicemic Plague

- Probably caused by direct deposition of the bacillus to the vasculature in the oral, tonsillar, and pharyngeal areas
- Sepsis without bubo formation (lymph nodes are bypassed in this form)
- Characteristics caused by disseminated intravascular coagulation (DIC) include aral cyanosis, ecchymosis, petechiae, and digital, penile, and nuchal gangrene
- Necrotic appendages and proximal purpuric lesions caused by endotoxemia

At the late septicemic shock stage, characteristics include elevated body temperature (up to 40.9°C or 105°F), tachycardia, tachypnea, and hypotension.

Differential Diagnosis

Bubonic Plague

- Acute adenitis (staphylococcal, streptococcal, tularemia)
- Cellulitis
- Enteric Gram-negative sepsis
- Lymphogranuloma venereum (LVG)
- Meningococcemia
- Rickettsiosis
- Syphilis

Pneumonic Plague

- Anthrax
- Brucellosis
- Malaria
- Staphylococcal enterotoxin B (SEB)
- Tularemia

Septicemic Plague

- Septicemia
- Septic shock
- Systemic inflammatory response syndrome

Laboratory Tests

- CBC: white blood count (WBC) elevated to 20,000 or greater; left shift is noted; WBC may be low in late septicemia
- Urinalysis: gross hematuria; red blood count (RBC) casts; proteinuria
- Arterial blood gas: possible hypoxia and/or acidosis
- Microscopy: smears from lymph node (bubo) aspirate, sputum, blood, or CSF
- Gram stain: Gram-negative pleomorphic coccobacilli
- Wright, Giemsa, and Wayson's stains also useful; bipolar "safety-pin" structure
- Definitive diagnosis relies on culturing bacteria from blood, sputum, CSF, or bubo aspirates:
  - *Slow growth: > 48 hours before cultures can be definitively identified*
  - *Optimal growth at 28°C*
  - *Blood and bubo cultures positive in majority of patients (> 85%)*
  - *Sputum cultures positive only if lung involvement present*
- Fluorescent antibody stain provides rapid diagnosis
- Fluorescent antibody titer: fourfold titer difference indicates infection
- PCR: insufficiently developed but very sensitive
- Laboratory procedures generating aerosols require Biosafety Level 3 containment; otherwise Biosafety Level 2 offers sufficient protection

Treatment

Plague is almost always fatal unless treatment is initiated within 24 hours of the onset of symptoms. The following antibiotics may be used:

- Streptomycin (30 mg/kg/day IM divided bid/qid, not to exceed 2g/day)
- Gentamicin (5 mg/kg/day IM or IV or 2 mg/kg loading dose followed by 1.75 mg/kg IM or IV q 8 hours)
- Doxycycline (200 mg initially then 100 mg q 12 hours)
- Ciprofloxacin may be effective but studies have only been conducted in animals (recommended regimen is 400 mg IV bid)
- Chloramphenicol required for treatment of plague meningitis (25 mg/kg IV loading dose, then 15 mg/kg IV qid) for 10 to 14 days. Patient usually afebrile in 3 to 4 days

Supportive treatment is usually required. At the early stages, administration of crystalloids and monitoring of vital signs, urine output, and general clinical state may be sufficient. Septic shock requires invasive hemodynamic monitoring, administration of crystalloids, and vasopressive agents. Intubation and mechanical ventilation with positive end-expiratory pressure (PEEP) may be needed.

Prophylaxis

- No vaccine available
- Doxycycline 100 mg PO bid (choice)
- Ciprofloxacin 500 mg PO bid (experimental)
- Tetracycline 250 mg PO qid
- Chloramphenicol 25 mg/kg PO qid

FACE-TO-FACE CONTACT (WITHIN 2 FEET) OF A HEALTHCARE PROVIDER WITH A PATIENT SUFFERING FROM PNEUMONIC PLAGUE OR EXPOSURE TO PLAGUE AEROSOL AS A RESULT OF TERRORISM OR WAR WARRANTS PROPHYLAXIS WITH ANTIBIOTICS FOR 7 DAYS. IF FEVER OR COUGH OCCURS, STANDARD TREATMENT SHOULD BE STARTED IMMEDIATELY.

Precautionary Measures

Prehospital Measures

- Standard universal precautions: goggles, gloves, and gown
- Respiratory protection mandatory if respiratory symptoms are present

Hospital Measures

- If respiratory symptoms are present, **strict isolation with droplet precautionary measures for at least 72 hours of antibiotic therapy** or until sputum cultures are negative in confirmed cases
- In absence of respiratory symptoms, isolation for 48 hours or until purulent discharge from bubos ceases
- Biosafety Level 2 or 3 required; Level 3 if aerosolization is possible

Q FEVER

This zoonotic, endemic disease is caused by *Coxiella burnetti*. Contrary to other rickettsial diseases, Q fever is contracted by inhalation rather than tick bite. Cattle, sheep, goats, dogs, cats, and birds constitute natural reservoirs and do not develop the disease even if infected. The pathogens, with high concentrations in the placental tissues of the host, are released into the environment during birth and in milk, urine, and feces. Close contact with animals subjects farmers and slaughterhouse workers to high risks of infection.

Laboratory personnel working with the cultures of *C. burnetti* are also at risk. Q fever has worldwide distribution in acute and chronic forms. Only the acute form has immediate relevance in the context of biological terrorism.

Signs and Symptoms

Acute Form

- Incubation: 9 to 40 days (average 18 to 21 days)
- Presentation with influenza-like symptoms
  - *Fever*
  - *Severe headache*
  - *Myalgia*
  - *Cough*
  - *Pleuritic chest pain*
  - *Sweats*
  - *Chills*
  - *Nausea*
  - *Anorexia*
- Specific findings may be absent
- Chest x-ray abnormalities show as patchy infiltrates resembling viral or mycoplasmal pneumonia
- Acute hepatitis may develop in approximately 33% of patients; findings include fever, malaise, hepatomegaly, pain in the right upper quadrant, and occasional jaundice
- Aseptic meningitis is rare (1% of cases)

Chronic Form

- Infective endocarditis
- Congestive heart failure
- Splenomegaly

- Hepatitis
- Hepatomegaly
- Osteomyelitis
- Clubbing
- Patients developing Q fever endocarditis may have predisposing factors, e.g., preexisting valvular heart disease or a vascular prosthesis

Clinical Features

Acute Form

- Clinically indistinct disease that resembles other viral illnesses or atypical forms of pneumonia
- Chest x-ray: variable, normal to widespread pneumonitis
- Need for differentiation from pneumonia caused by:
  – *Mycoplasma pneumoniae*
  – *Legionella pneumophila*
  – *Chlamydia psittaci*
  – *Chlamydia pneumoniae*
- Diagnosis confirmed serologically
- Hepatic ultrasound may detect granulomatous hepatitis

One strong indicator of the possibility for a large scale exposure to aerosolized Q fever bacilli is provided by significant numbers of people from the same geographic area who present within a relatively brief period (7 to 14 days) with nonspecific febrile illness associated with pulmonary symptoms in approximately 25% of all cases.

Chronic Form

- Endocarditis of aortic valve common
- Granulomatous hepatitis

Laboratory Tests

Acute Form

- CBC: normal in 70% of cases; WBC elevated in the remainder
- Slight elevation of transaminases (×2 to 3); bilirubin normal in liver function tests

- Serologic testing not helpful acutely
- Chest x-ray: normal to widespread pneumonitis

At later stages, providing a baseline has been established, a four-fold increase in complement-fixing antibody titer against phase II antigen approximately 3 to 4 weeks after the onset may be helpful in establishing definitive diagnosis.

Chronic Form

- Serology: complement fixing antibody titer against phase I antigen ≥1:200 or IgG ≥ II titer indicates infection
- Culture: negative endocarditis
- Liver biopsy: granulomas
- Cerebrospinal fluid consistent with aseptic meningitis: elevated WBC with mainly monocytes, elevated protein, normal glucose, negative Gram stain
- Hepatic ultrasound may reveal granulomatous hepatitis
- Echocardiogram: endocarditis of the aortic valve hepatic ultrasound most common; prosthetic valves may be affected

Differential Diagnosis

- Legionnaires' disease
- Mononucleosis
- Other tick-borne fevers
- Plague
- Pneumonia (mycoplasmic, viral)
- Tularemia

Treatment

Acute Form

Although eventual spontaneous resolution is very likely, all patients must be treated in order to reduce the risk of subsequent complications.

- Tetracycline 500 mg q 6 hours
- Doxycycline 100 mg q 12 hours for 5 to 7 days
- Ciprofloxacin (experimental data only)

Chronic Form

- Treatment of Q fever endocarditis is difficult
- Tetracycline, doxycycline (in combination with TMP/SMX), rifampin for 12 months or longer may produce results; valve replacement may be ultimately necessary

Prophylaxis

- Vaccine is available in the U.S. only for at-risk personnel and for research purposes
- Vaccination of immune individuals may result in severe local reactions
- Tetracycline 500 mg q 6 hours for 5 to 7 days effective when given 8 to 12 days after exposure
- Doxycycline 100 mg q 12 hours for 5 to 7 days effective when given 8 to 12 days after exposure
- Chemoprophylaxis may be ineffective and prolong disease when given immediately (1 to 7 days) after exposure to *C. burnetti*

Precautionary Measures

C. burnetti is extremely virulent (a single organism may cause infection) and resistant to inactivation. It can survive for long periods in dust and feces particles. Standard universal precautions should be observed. One documented case of person-to-person transmission exists. Laboratory outbreaks have been reported.

The risk of serious complications accompanying the chronic form of the disease and the extreme virulence of the bacillus suggest enhanced vigilance in contacts with animals in areas where Q fever has been reported. This applies also to handling contaminated samples in clinical and laboratory settings.

TULAREMIA

This zoonotic disease (known also as rabbit or deer fly fever) is caused by *Francisella tularensis,* a small Gram-negative, aerobic coccobacillus. The disease is common in western south central U.S. and is acquired by humans through contact with body fluids of infected animals or through tick, deer fly, or mosquito bites. Infection via inhalation of contaminated dust or ingestion of foods containing bacteria is less common.

Tularemia bacilli may remain viable for weeks in water, soil, hides, and carcasses. In frozen rabbit meat, they remain virulent even after years of storage. The bacilli are resistant to temperatures below freezing, but heat and disinfectants kill them easily. Six clinical forms are reported in man. The virulence is high; as few as 10 to 25 organisms (subcutaneous or inhalational exposure) are sufficient to produce clinical disease. Mortality may reach 30% in untreated patients.

A large number of patients presenting with similar systemic illness and nonproductive pneumonia within a short time (7 to 14 days) may be indicators of a bioterrorist event.

Signs and Symptoms

General Symptoms

- Incubation 1 to 21 days; typical incubation is 3 to 5 days
- Males affected more frequently than females
- Bimodal prevalence, probably related to specific activities:
  - *Children — May through August*
  - *Adults — December and January*
- Abrupt, often severe onset
- Symptoms last for a few days and recur after brief remission
- Symptoms common to all forms include:
  - *Fever*
  - *Chills*
  - *Malaise*
  - *Fatigue*
  - *Prostration*
  - *Headache*
  - *Myalgia*
  - *Cough (nonproductive)*
  - *Substernal discomfort*
  - *Pharyngitis*
  - *Vomiting*
  - *Abdominal pain*

Clinical Features

Ulceroglandular Form (75 to 85% of Cases)

- Predominantly affects adults
- Small erythomatous papula at inoculation site on skin or mucous membrane; papula enlarges and ulcerates within 2 to 3 days
- Rabbit-associated tularemia affects hands and fingers; may involve axillary or epitrochlear adenopathy
- Tick-associated tularemia affects groin and lower extremities; may involve inguinal or femoral adenopathy
- Systemic adenopathy may occur
- Ulcers are painful, characterized by raised edges and jagged floors

Glandular Form (5 to 20% of Cases)

- Fever
- Tender lymphadenopathy
- No skin ulcers

Oculoglandular Form (1 to 5% of Cases)

- Conjunctival inoculation secondary to touching or rubbing eyes with contaminated hands, aerosol exposure, or splatter with body fluids
- Unilateral, purulent, and painful conjunctivitis
- Painful cervical (most common), preauricular, or submandibular lymphadenopathy
- Photophobia
- Lachrymosis
- Lid edema

Oropharyngeal Form (<12% of Cases)

- Secondary to ingestion of undercooked, contaminated meat
- Exudative pharyngitis or tonsillitis
- Cervical lymphadenopathy
- Abdominal pain
- Nausea and vomiting
- Diarrhea
- Occasional gastrointestinal bleeding

Pneumonic Form (7 to 20% of Cases)

- Primary infection through ingestion or inhalation of organisms in water or dust; secondary after hematogenous or septicemic invasion
- Nonproductive cough
- Dyspnea

Typhoidal Form (5 to 30% of Cases)

- Primary infection after aerosol inhalation
- Onset severe and fulminant
- Systemic; no obvious source of entry; may ensue via infection routes of other forms
- **Lymphadenopathy absent**; may make definitive clinical diagnosis difficult
- All other symptoms listed for other forms may be present

Differential Diagnosis

Typhoidal Syndromes

- Malaria
- Rickettsia
- Salmonella

Pneumonic Pathologies

- Anthrax
- Brucellosis
- Diphtheria
- Mycoplasmal infections
- Parainfluenza virus
- Plague
- Pneumonia
- Q fever
- SEB

Laboratory Tests

- Chest x-rays indicated for all patients with suspected tularemia

■ Chest x-ray findings in tularemia pneumonia include:
  – *Bilateral patchy infiltrates*
  – *Lobar infiltrates*
  – *Cavity lesions*
  – *Pleural effusion*
■ Standard (nonspecific) blood test results:
  – *Serum transaminase may be mildly elevated (≤50% of cases)*
  – *Serum lactic dehydrogenase mildly elevated*
  – *Serum alkaline phosphatase mildly elevated*
  – *Serum creatine kinase elevated (rhabdomyolysis)*
  – *WBC may be elevated; frequently within reference range*
  – *Mild thrombocytopenia*
  – *Hyponatremia observed occasionally*
  – *Cerebrospinal fluid usually normal; mild elevation of proteins or pleocytosis may be present*
■ Blood culture:
  – *Poor sensitivity*
  – *Best cultured on media containing cysteine (glucose cysteine blood agar)*
■ Serology:
  – *Antibodies measured by agglutination or ELISA*
  – *Agglutination titer: >1:160 presumptively positive; treatment may be started*
  – *Antibodies in sufficient levels for confident diagnosis 2 weeks after infection*
  – *Second titer with a fourfold increase after 2 weeks confirms diagnosis*
  – *Earlier titers may be negative*

Treatment

■ Course of treatment for all drugs is 10 to 14 days
  – *Streptomycin considered agent of choice (7.5 to 10 mg/kg IM q 12 hours)*
  – *Ciprofloxacin (400 mg IV q 12 hours); after clinical improvement, oral administration (500 mg q 12 hours)*
  – *Ciprofloxacin (750 mg PO q 12 hours)*
  – *Gentamycin (3 to 5 mg/kg/day IV divided q 6 to 8 hours **or** 5mg/kg IV qd)*

A streptomycin-resistant strain of *F. tularensis* represents the potential choice for bioterrorist applications. It is sensitive to gentamycin. Compared to streptomycin, gentamycin affects a broader spectrum of Gram-negative bacteria and may be the agent of choice when tularemia diagnosis is considered but uncertain.

Prophylaxis

- Experimental vaccine exists
- No immunoprophylaxis
- Preexposure prophylaxis: agents given for anthrax and plague may offer protection
- Postexposure prophylaxis when given within 24 hours following aerosol exposure:
  - *Ciprofloxacin (500 mg PO q 12 hours)*
  - *Doxycycline (100 mg PO q 12 hours)*
  - *Tetracycline (500 mg PO q 12 hours)*
- Treatment course: 14 days
- Chemoprophylaxis is not recommended for natural exposures (ticks, rabbits, flies, etc.)

Precautionary Measures

Interperson transmission is rare, but cases have been reported among laboratory personnel. Due to the very infectious character of the bacillus in aerosolized form, laboratory work involving cultures of *F. tularensis* must be performed at Biosafety Level 3. In-hospital precautions require standard measures of protection, but the possibility of infection through contact with contaminated body fluids, clothing, etc., must be borne in mind. Isolation is not required.

VIRAL DISEASES

EQUINE ENCEPHALOMYELITIS

Equine encephalomyelitis describes three discrete forms of zoonotic viral infections initially presenting as nonspecific febrile illnesses known as Venezuelan, Eastern, and Western equine encephalomyelitis (VEE, EEE, and WEE.) **The viruses are endemic in northern South America and Trinidad and cause rare cases of human encephalitis in northern Central America, Mexico, and Florida.** The three viruses responsible for equine encephalomyelitis belong to the genus *Alphaviridae* (fam. Togoviridae) endemic to the Americas. Several other pathogens belonging to the same genus are known in other parts of the world and cause an acute febrile illness syndrome often associated with severe polyarthritic elements (viruses from the Togoviridae family cause diseases with different manifestations, e.g., rubella).

Laboratory manipulations (including genetic changes) of alphaviruses are relatively easy and alphaviruses have served frequently as models in studies of viral biology. Moreover, production of large quantities of these viruses does not require highly sophisticated facilities because they replicate rapidly, store easily, readily adapt to dissimilar hosts, and can be aerosolized with little difficulty. **They can be used readily as bioterrorist weapons, especially because their environmental concentrations that produce significant infection rates need not be as high as those of many other pathogens**.

Aerosol release would be the most likely form of a bioterrorist attack employing an equine encephalitis virus (EEV). Equine encephalitis is usually nonlethal (<1% overall mortality), and an epidemic resulting from a bioterrorist attack has the potential of causing a large-scale disease outbreak. Significant psychological stress of the population, interruption of normal activities, and severe economical disturbances would be the primary consequences of terrorism-associated release of EEV.

Natural infections in humans and horses are acquired through mosquito bites (*Culex, Mansonia, Psorophora,* and *Aedes* species), although bats, birds, rodents, and equines (horses, donkeys, and mules) constitute other natural reservoirs of the disease. Humans acquire the disease as accidental inclusions in the animal–mosquito–animal cycle. **However, person-to-person infection appears possible.**

Neurotropism and severity of neurological complications are markedly different among viruses causing encephalitic fevers. Upon initial presentation, all forms of encephalitic fevers manifest as systemic viral febrile syndromes. Specific diagnosis may be difficult and the possibility of misdiagnosis is great.

THE APPEARANCE OF VEE, EEE, AND WEE OUTSIDE THEIR GEO-GRAPHICAL RANGES INDICATES THE POSSIBILITY OF A BIOTER-RORIST ATTACK. THE INCIDENCE OF SEVERE INFECTIONS WOULD BE SIGNIFICANTLY HIGHER IF AN AEROSOLIZED VIRUS SERVED AS A BIOTERRORIST WEAPON DUE TO DIRECT INFECTION OF THE OLFACTORY NERVE AND SUBSEQUENT RAPID MIGRATION TO THE CENTRAL NERVOUS SYSTEM.

Signs and Symptoms (General)

- Most VEE infections are mild; EEE and WEE are predominant
- Malaise
- Fever
- Severe headache
- Confusion
- Rigor
- Photophobia
- Myalgia

Venezuelan Equine Encephalitis

Signs and Symptoms

- Incubation period: 1 to 6 days
- All infections are symptomatic; only a low percentage show central nervous system involvement
- Patients may be incapacitated 7 to 14 days
- Malaise
- Chills
- Sore throat and cough
- Muscle tenderness
- Nausea and vomiting

Clinical Features

- High fever (38 to 40.5°C)
- Photophobia
- Conjunctival infection
- Erythematous pharynx
- Myalgia of legs and lumbosacral region

- Mild central nervous system involvement:
  - *Lethargy*
  - *Somnolence*
  - *Mild confusion*
  - *Possible nuchal rigidity*
  - *Possible hypotension in dehydrated patients*
- Severe central nervous system involvement:
  - *Seizures*
  - *Ataxia*
  - *Paralysis*
- Mortality (severe infection): 10% in adults, ≤35% in children

Differential Diagnosis

- Encephalitis
- Malaria
- Meningitis
- West Nile fever

Laboratory Tests

- During first 3 days of infection, striking leukopenia, lymphopenia, and thrombocytopenia
- Definitive diagnosis only by virus isolation, serology, and polymerase chain reaction

Eastern Equine Encephalitis (EEE)

- Natural habitat: swamps and forests
- Onset in children is more sudden
- Fatality rate highest in children and the elderly

Signs and Symptoms

- Incubation period: 5 to 15 days
- Febrile prodrome up to 11 days before onset of neurological symptoms
- Viremia develops during prodrome; may remain undetectable when signs of clinical encephalitis appear

Clinical Features

- Rapid onset of high fever
- Stiff neck
- Vomiting
- Drowsiness
- Elevated opening pressure during lumbar puncture
- Neurological features include:
  - *Motor involvement with pareses*
  - *Disturbances of autonomous functions*
  - *Excessive salivation*
  - *Disturbances of respiratory regulation*
  - *Nervous system: ≤30% of survivors show seizures, spastic paralysis, and cognitive impairment ranging from mild to severe dementia*

Differential Diagnosis

- Other encephalitic fevers
- Brain abscess
- Central nervous system trauma
- Catscratch disease
- Ehrlichiosis
- Herpes simplex encephalitis
- Hypoglycemia
- Intracranial tumor
- Meningitis
- Status epilepticus
- Subarachnoid hemorrhage
- Toxoplasmosis
- Tuberculosis

Laboratory Tests

- Early leukopenia followed by leukocytosis
- Cerebrospinal fluid: leukocytic pleocytosis, particularly in children (>1000 mononuclear cells/μl)
- Definitive diagnosis only by virus isolation, serology, and polymerase chain reaction

Western Equine Encephalitis (WEE)

Infants and elderly are particularly vulnerable (≤10% mortality rate).

Signs and Symptoms

- Incubation period: 5 to 10 days
- Malaise
- Headache
- Fever
- Nausea and vomiting
- Gradual worsening of symptoms accompanied by somnolence that may progress to delirium and coma
- Most severely affected patients die in ≤7 days
- Long recovery periods characterized by:
  - *Fatigue*
  - *Recurrent headaches*
  - *Impaired concentration*
  - *Emotional lability*
  - *Permanent motor weakness, cognitive deficits, and seizure disorders in some patients*

Differential Diagnosis

- Other encephalitic fevers
- Brain abscess
- Central nervous system trauma
- Catscratch disease
- Ehrlichiosis
- Herpes simplex encephalitis
- Hypoglycemia
- Intracranial tumor
- Meningitis
- Status epilepticus
- Subarachnoid hemorrhage
- Toxoplasmosis
- Tuberculosis

Clinical Features

- Nuchal rigidity
- Impaired mental acuity
- Upper motor neuron deficits
- Abnormal reflexes

Laboratory Tests

- Viremia rarely detectable in patients with encephalitic symptoms
- Lymphocytic pleocytosis (10 to 400 mononuclear cells/μl)
- Virus can be isolated from throat swabs in initial 2 days of illness

Equine Encephalitis Virus Identification

- Time consuming; may be performed only in Biosafety Level 3 laboratories
- Inoculation of cell culture or suckling mice with serum or throat swab specimens using Gold Standard Assay for VEE

Serology

- IgM ELISA
- IgG ELISA
- Hemagglutination inhibition
- Complement fixation

In patients without known prior exposure to VEE, diagnosis is confirmed by identifying IgM antibodies in a single sample taken 5 to 7 days after the onset of the disease.

Treatment

- No specific therapy
- Supportive treatment in patients with uncomplicated disease; analgesics to relieve headache and myalgia
- In clinical encephalitis patients, specialized treatment involving anticonvulsants, fluid and electrolyte balance support, and airway maintenance may be required

Prophylaxis

- Two investigational vaccines available:
  - *TC-83 (licensed for Equide), 0.5 ml SC. Subsequent susceptibility to clinical infection unknown. The vaccine causes moderate to severe side effects (headache, fever, malaise) in ≤20% of cases. Counterindicated during pregnancy and ongoing clinical infection*

– *TC-84 (not for primary immunization; used as a booster for TC-83 nonresponders), 0.5 ml SC*
■ Immunoprophylaxis: no pre- or postexposure prophylaxis available
■ Chemoprophylaxis: experimental; combined with α-interferon or polyICLC provides effective postexposure prophylaxis in animals. No human data available

Precautionary Measures

VEE has been isolated from throat washings of infected patients, and aerosol transmissions in laboratories have been reported. While standard precautions appear adequate, vector control is important in areas where mosquitoes are common. Generally, patients should be housed in screened rooms treated persistently with insecticide during the febrile and immediately postfebrile (at least 72 hours) stages. Standard disinfectants or temperature ≥80°C for 30 minutes will kill the virus.

VIRAL HEMORRHAGIC FEVERS (VHFS)

Viral hemorrhagic fevers are caused by a group of taxonomically different RNA viruses. All pose natural threats of infection, although the regions of where they are endemic may be confined to well-defined geographical territories. Under normal conditions, infection of humans occurs through contacts with infected animals or insect vectors. Four families, Arenaviridae, Bunyaviridae, Filoviridae, and Flaviviridae, although taxonomically diverse, are the primary causes of hemorrhagic fevers. The viruses are extremely pathogenic and, although relatively stable in aerosol form, are susceptible to detergents and household bleach. Their ability to replicate in cell cultures and their resulting yields make them potentially lethal as bioterrorist agents, particularly when introduced into ventilation systems.

The clinical syndrome caused by these viruses is generally known as VHF (viral hemorrhagic fever). Its dominant clinical features are consequences of microvascular damage and pathological changes in the permeability of the microvascular bed.

Arenaviridae

- Lassa fever (West Africa)
- Junin (Argentine) fever
- Machupo (Bolivian) fever
- Sabia (Brazilian) fever
- Guanarito (Venezuelan) fever

Small rodents constitute their chief reservoirs. Infection occurs typically through inhalation of dust contaminated with rodent excreta. One case of Sabia infection at a U.S. laboratory has been described. It is estimated that in West Africa up to 300,000 cases of Lassa fever may occur over the next 10 years, with approximately 5,000 deaths resulting from the infection.

Bunyaviridae

- Rift Valley fever (Phlebovirus)
- Crimean–Congo fever (Nairovirus)
- Hemorrhagic fever with renal syndrome (HFRS) (Hantavirus)

Each family has a different vector (Phlebovirus — mosquitoes; Nairovirus — ticks; Hantavirus — rodents and their excreta). The highly infectious Crimean–Congo virus has been particularly troublesome by causing aerosol-mediated nosocomial outbreaks in Africa, Asia, and Europe. The cause of a 1993 U.S. outbreak of Hantavirus cardiopulmonary syndrome (HCPS) was the result of infection with the Sin Nombre (without name) virus.

Filoviridae

- Ebola fever
- Marburg fever

Little is known about the natural histories of these viruses. Ebola–Zaire is associated with 90% mortality, and Ebola–Sudan with 50%. In both cases, serologically different viral strains have been identified. The only known outbreak of Ebola in the U.S. (caused by a different strain) took place at an animal facility in Reston, VA. Although hundreds of the infected monkeys died, no cases of human infection were caused by what is now known as the Ebola–Reston virus. Human infections with the Marburg virus are more sporadic and a total of five occurrences have been reported in Africa, Germany (Marburg), and Yugoslavia.

Flaviviridae

- Yellow fever
- Dengue fever
- Kyasanur forest fever
- Omsk fever

Mosquitoes are the vectors of dengue and yellow fevers, and ticks are the carriers of Kyasanur and Omsk fevers. **Dengue fever is not infectious by the aerosol route**.

Signs and Symptoms

NOTE: Travel to areas where the responsible viruses are known to occur, professional involvement (laboratory personnel), or biological warfare threat are particularly strong indicators of possible VHF infection.

Initial Symptoms

- Fever
- Myalgia
- Headache
- Fatigue
- Abdominal pain
- Prostration

Advanced Stage Symptoms

- Petechiae
- Hematemesis
- Bloody diarrhea
- Generalized mucous membrane hemorrhage
- Hypotension
- Renal insufficiency (proportional to cardiovascular compromise)
- Altered mental state
- Shock

Clinical Features

General Features

VHF should be suspected in all patients presenting with severe febrile illness and evidence of vascular involvement:

- Fever
- Pharyngitis
- Postural hypotension
- Petechiae
- Flushing of face and chest
- Conjunctival infection
- Nondependent edema
- Gastrointestinal bleeding
- Photophobia
- Neurological involvement (hyperesthesia, dizziness, confusion, and tremors)

Table 3.1 Overview of Symptoms Characterizing Hemorrhagic Fevers Relevant to Bioterrorism

Feature	Disease
Jaundice and other features of hepatitis	Crimean-Congo fever; Rift Valley fever (occasional); yellow fever (jaundice indicates poor prognosis); Ebola fever; Marburg fever
Diagnostically significant maculo-papular rash (profound disseminated intravascular coagulation of DIC)	Ebola, Marburg
Very severe hemorrhage (DIC); flushes on head, neck, and upper back may have diagnostic significance	Crimean-Congo
Hemorrhages	Guanarito; Junin; Machupo; Sabia
Uncommon hemorrhages	Rift Valley
Absence of cutaneous signs of vascular instability	Rift Valley
No hemorrhages	Lassa fever; Hantavirus; Sin Nombre
Very severe peripheral edema	Lassa
Pulmonary involvement	Kyanasur; Omsk
Pulmonary failure (Hantavirus pulmonary syndrome or HPS)	Hantavirus; Sin Nombre
Renal failure	Hantavirus
Retinitis	Rift Valley
Hearing Loss	Lassa fever
Positive Tourniquet test	Dengue
Nocosomial transmission	Crimean-Congo

Note: Not all symptoms may be seen upon presentation. Some are characteristic of the early stages of illness. Others appear later. The chart clearly indicates that many of the diseases may be easily misdiagnosed as ill-defined febrile syndromes. Only the subsequent progress of the infection will reveal its characteristic landmarks. It is essential that during periods of heightened terrorism alerts, all healthcare personnel are vigilant to atypical presentations of otherwise common diseases. A list of diseases that should be considered as a part of differential diagnosis is provided.

Disease-Specific Features

Rift Valley and yellow fever viruses are primarily hepatotrophic. With the exception of Lassa, where it is rare and found only in the most severe cases, neurologic involvement is common.

Differential Diagnosis

- Disseminated intravascular coagulation (DIC)
- Hemolytic uremic syndrome
- Leptospirosis
- Malaria
- Meningococcemia
- Rickettsial infection
- Salmonella infection
- Shigellosis
- Thrombocytopenic purpura
- Typhoid fever

Laboratory Tests

Blood

- CBC: thrombocytopenia and leukopenia **except** in Lassa, Hanta and very severe Crimean-Congo hemorrhagic fevers
- Aspartate aminotransferase (AST) correlates with the severity of Lassa hemorrhagic fever

Urine

- Proteinuria and hematuria are common
- Their absence rules out Argentine, Bolivian, and Hanta hemorrhagic fevers

Virology

- Definitive diagnosis based on virological testing
- ELISA detects IgM antibodies during the acute illness in Argentine, Crimean-Congo, Lassa, and Rift Valley hemorrhagic fevers and yellow fever
- Virus cultures may take 3 to 10 days; longer for Hantavirus
- Reverse transcriptase polymerase chain reaction (RT–PCR) can be safely performed following chloroform/methanol extraction
- RT-PCR is suitable for real-time virus identification when isolation of virus is impractical

EXTREME precautions must be taken during sampling, handling, and packaging of all samples from infected patients. Testing should be conducted either at CDC facilities in Atlanta or at the U.S. Army Medical Research Institute of Infectious Diseases (USMRIID) at Ft. Detrick, MD, which has the required maximum containment facilities (BL-4).

Treatment

General Measures

- Only critical or intensive care will save seriously ill patients
- **Avoid air transportation if possible** because pressure changes may affect lung–water balance
- Supportive measures with careful use of sedatives and analgesics in management of restlessness, myalgia, and hyperesthesia
- Avoid immunosuppressants (e.g., steroids)
- Do not administer IM injections, aspirin, or agents with anticoagulant properties
- Secondary infections are common
- **Unless clearly indicated,** avoid IV lines, in-dwelling catheters, and invasive procedures

Control of Hemorrhages

- Treatment of minor bleeding should not be attempted unless hemorrhagic fever is definitively excluded
- Treatment of major hemorrhages remains controversial; no controlled study results are available. Field observations indicate the effectiveness of vigorous administration of:
  - *Heparin to prevent DIS; administer early*
  - *Fresh frozen plasma*
  - *Clotting factor concentrates*
  - *Platelets*

Hypotension and Shock

- Cautious administration of colloid or crystalloid fluids; possibility of pulmonary edema and myocardial complications due to increased vascular permeability
- Dopamine (5 to 10 μg/kg/minute IV) suggested for patients unresponsive to fluid replacement
- Dengue hemorrhagic fever: due to systemic capillary leakage syndrome:
  - *Use crystalloid fluids infused through a large-bore cannula*

  - *Infusion rate >>30 ml/hour (adults)*
  - *If no response, follow with albumin*
- Hanta hemorrhagic fever: due to possible renal failure and polyuria during recovery:
  - *Careful fluid and electrolyte management necessary*
  - *Renal dialysis may be needed*

Drug Treatment

- Ribavarin (30 mg/kg IV followed by 15 mg/kg q 6 hours for 4 days, followed by 7.5 mg/kg q 8 hours for 6 days)
- Treatment is most effective if begun within 7 days of onset
- Lower IV doses or 2.0 g PO followed by 1.0 g PO for 10 days may be useful
- Ribavarin treatment useful for Crimean–Congo, Hanta (if started within 4 days of onset), Lassa, and Rift Valley hemorrhagic fevers
  - *Ribavarin treatment is ineffective for Ebola and Marburg hemorrhagic fevers*
  - *For flaviviridae infections (dengue, Kyasanur, and Omsk hemorrhagic fevers and yellow fever)*

Prophylaxis

A vaccine against yellow fever (mandatory for travelers to endemic regions of Africa and South America) is available. An experimental vaccine (Candid #1) is available against Argentina hemorrhagic fever. Vaccines against dengue and Hantaviruses are in early stages of testing.

Precautionary Measures

With the exception of dengue that poses no secondary infection danger, and patients infected with Hanta virus but showing no evidence of viral presence in the blood or exreta at the time of clinical presentation, all other viral hemorrhagic fever patients have very significant levels of viruses in their blood, saliva, and other secretions. **All potential sources of exposure — needles, blades, instruments, etc. — must be handled with extreme care. Nosocomial infections caused by Crimean–Congo virus with secondary spread of the disease among the emergency and operating room staff have been documented.**

Crimean–Congo, Ebola, Lassa, and Marburg hemorrhagic fever viruses may be spread nocosomially via aerosol dispersion. A patient with suspected hemorrhagic fever should be isolated in a private room, if possible, with negative air pressure inside from the outset (to avoid subsequent transportation to other patients' rooms). An adjacent room should be made available as a lock space and for storage, decontamination, and donning and removing protective barriers. **All personnel entering the patient room must wear gloves, gowns, surgical masks, and face shields. If severe coughing, diarrhea, vomiting, or hemorrhage is present, respiratory protection should be upgraded to at least HEPA filtered mask level. An air purifying respirator or positive pressure respirator may be considered. If large amounts of blood and excreta are on the floor, shoe and leg coverings should be worn.**

Before leaving a patient's room, healthcare personnal should discard protective barriers and thoroughly clean shoes with gloved hands before entering the anteroom. All specimens collected for laboratory analysis must be placed in double bags, sealed, and surface-decontaminated prior to transport to the laboratory.

Local laboratory personnel handling viral hemorrhagic fever specimens should also exercise extreme precautionary measures. They should work in biosafety cabinets, and use complete contact and respiratory protection.

Handling of the dead patients should be reduced to the absolute minimum. Bodies should be sealed in leak-proof bags and either buried or cremated as soon as possible.

While overreaction in dealing with viral hemorrhagic fever patients may occur and is understandable, it may have a negative impact on patients and staff. On the other hand, the extreme virulence of the pathogens that cause viral hemorrhagic fevers dictates the necessity for maximum reasonable measures to prevent secondary infections. **Such precautions include autoclaving or liquid decontamination (with hypochlorite or phenol disinfectants) of excreta and all other contaminated items.**

SMALLPOX

The most notorious member of the Poxviridae family, variola, occurs in at least two viral strains — variola minor and variola major. Apart from serving as a major cause of large-scale mortality, variola also has the distinction of being one of the most historically significant biological weapons. The Spanish were alleged to have used it as early as the 15th century during their conquest of the Americas. The British used smallpox in the French and Indian Wars in the late 18th century. In both cases, smallpox was directed at a native population that had no immunity against the disease. Smallpox was weaponized during World War II by the Unit 731 of the Imperial Japanese Army.

From a medical point of view, the discovery by Edward Jennings that cowpox infection provides immunity against smallpox is probably more significant through its introduction of the concept of vaccination. Interestingly, George Washington ordered cowpox inoculation of all of the Revolutionary troops as a protection against smallpox.

The World Health Organization declared officially in 1980 that smallpox was eradicated as a health threat. However, both Russia and the U.S. maintain repositories of variola virus at Vector Laboratories and the Centers for Disease Control, respectively. The issue of whether these stocks should be eliminated is hotly debated. Nonetheless, the possibility of reintroduction of variola via natural or artificial routes is real. Because the gene sequence of variola is available and because variola shows significant homology with other Orthopoxviridae, intentional engineering of the virus by a hostile entity is possible. Weaponization is facilitated by the considerable stability of the virus in aerosol form.

Variola major is the predominant source of mortality (30% of infected cases). The significantly milder variola minor (alastrim) is associated with a fatality rate of ≤1%. In addition to the two common forms, two rare varieties — **hemorrhagic** and **malignant** — have been described. **In hemorrhagic smallpox, the rash is accompanied by hemorrhage into the mucous membranes and skin. In the malignant variety, the lesions do not progress to the pustular stage but remain soft and flat. Both forms are invariably fatal.**

Vaccinia, cowpox, and monkeypox are caused by other members of the Orthopoxviridaem but only smallpox is transmitted from person to person. Although manifestations of vaccinia, cowpox, and monkeypox are generally similar to those of smallpox, their clinical courses are significantly milder.

The natural incidence of smallpox follows temporal sequence of chickenpox and measles, with the number of reported cases peaking during winter and early spring. Significant weakening of immunity against smallpox and cessation of immunizations during the last two decades mean that the age distribution of infections during a U.S. outbreak would likely be similar to the incidence reported in the general population worldwide.

Implantation of the virus in the oropharyngeal or respiratory muscosal membranes initiates the infection. Although the size of the infective dose is unknown, smallpox is extremely contagious; a few viral particles are necessary to initiate infection. **The disease spreads through person-to-person contact. Contaminated clothing, bedding, etc., constitute viral reservoirs. Insect or animal vectors or reservoirs are unknown.**

Signs and Symptoms

- Incubation period: 12 to 14 days (range is 7 to 19 days); **no viral shedding observed during incubation period**
- Following incubation period, a sudden onset prodrome with influenza-like symptoms:
  - *Fever*
  - *Malaise*
  - *Prostration*
  - *Severe back pain*
  - *Vomiting*
  - *Abdominal pain (rare)*
  - *Delirium (15%)*
  - *Erythematous rash in light-skinned patients (10%)*
- Patients are most infectious during the prodrome stage lasting 2 to 4 days
- Prodrome is followed by the reduction of fever and appearance of rash on the face, hands, and forearms
- Development of characteristic lesions (7 to 10 days):
  - *First lesions in oral mucosa*
  - *Mucosal lesions facilitate release of virus particles during coughing and sneezing*
  - *Centrifugal distribution of skin lesions. The density is significantly greater on the face and extremities than on trunk* **(CHARACTERISTIC diagnostic feature)**
  - *Axillae, palms, soles, and antecubital areas spared from lesions.*
  - **Synchronous** *(all at the same stage) lesion development* **(CHARACTERISTIC diagnostic feature)**
  - *Maculae > papulae > vesicles > pustules;* **contents are highly infectious**
- Fever may reappear approximately 7 days after onset of rash
- Scabs form 8 to 14 days after onset; scabs contain active virus particles

Clinical Features

- Smallpox — **centrifugal lesions**; varicella (chickenpox) — centripetal lesions
- Smallpox — **synchronous lesions**; varicella — asynchronous lesions
- Smallpox — **firm, deep papulae**; varicella — soft, superficial papulae
- Smallpox — **scabs form 10 to 14 days after onset of rash**; varicella — scabs form 4 to 7 days after onset of rash
- Smallpox — **scars**; varicella — no scars
- Smallpox — **fever**; varicella — minimal fever or none
- Lymphadenopathy more common in **monkeypox**

Differential Diagnosis

- Erythema multiforme
- Malignant measles
- Meningococcemia
- Monkeypox
- Secondary syphilis
- Typhus
- Varicella (chickenpox)

Laboratory Tests

- Presence of virions demonstrated by electron microscopy
- Light microscopy:
  - *Giemsa stain: aggregations of variola virus particles (Guarnieri bodies) showing as reddish, hematoxylinophyllic inclusions in the cytoplasms of cells from vesicular scrapings*
  - *Gispen modified silver stain: black cytoplasmic inclusions*
- Standard laboratory tests do not distinguish variola, monkeypox, or cowpox
- Lumbar puncture in **hemorrhagic variola** to exclude possibility of meningococcemia
- Polymerase chain reaction required for definitive diagnosis

Treatment

No specific treatment available.

Management (<3 Days Postexposure)

- Standard vaccine
  - *Vaccinia immune globulin (VIG) (0.6 ml/kg IM):*
  - *Provides less than 70% protection when given early during the incubation period*
  - *Due to the large volume that must be injected (~42 ml/70 kg body weight), injections must be given at multiple sites over 24- to 36-hour period*
- VIG is indicated for treatment of complications resulting from inoculation with vaccinia vaccine

Management (>3 Days Postexposure)

- Smallpox vaccine and VIG are recommended
- Cidofovir protective in animal studies; no human data available
- Hydration to prevent fluid loss caused by fever and breakdown of the skin barrier
- Antibiotics to prevent secondary infection

Prophylaxis

- Vaccinia virus: strong cross-protection for 5 years; partial protection for 10 years
- Vaccination is strongly contraindicated for:
  - *Immunosuppressed patients*
  - *Patients with HIV*
  - *Patients with history or evidence of eczema*
  - *Partners and household members of patients with any of the above conditions*
  - *Pregnancy*
- Vaccination may result in complications:
  - *Progressive vaccinia (in immunosuppressed individuals — 75% fatality rate)*
  - *Eczema vaccinatum (in patients with history of eczema — <15% fatality rate)*
  - *Postvaccinal encephalitis seen after primary vaccination (25% mortality rate)*
  - *Generalized vaccinia (in immunosuppressed patients — good prognosis)*
  - *Autoinoculation to face, eyelids, genital area, or other persons*

Precautionary Measures

It is believed that each person infected with smallpox is likely to infect 20 others during the course of the illness. **STRICT ADEHERENCE TO PRECAUTIONARY MEASURES IS MANDATORY.**

Prehospital Measures

Strict universal precautions (blood, body fluids, droplets) must be observed by all emergency medical services personnel involved in prehospital handling and transport of a patient suspected of smallpox infection. Immediate vaccination and quarantine are mandatory.

Hospital Measures

- Immediate contact and droplet isolation
- Indirect transmission through contaminated clothing and bedding is unlikely but cannot be excluded
- Isolation of treating physicians and nursing staff may be considered
- Immediate notification of local public health authorities

Other Measures

Quarantine of all persons in contact with the index case for minimum of **17 days prior to the illness.**

If quarantine is impractical, isolation at home with a **daily body temperature check is advisable. SUDDEN ELEVATION OF TEMPERATURE ≥38°C (101°F) DURING 17 DAYS FOLLOWING CONTACT WITH THE INDEX CASE SUGGESTS SMALLPOX INFECTION.**

Decontamination

Under favorable conditions, aerosol-released variola virus may persist up to 24 hours. Hence, by the time first cases of infections are detected, the virus will be completely absent from the environment. In a hospital setting, likelihood of secondary (nosocomial) spread of the virus through contaminated bedding is likely. Indications suggest that the virus in clothing may remain viable for extended periods. **Careful double bagging during removal, followed by autoclaving and/or laundering in hot water and bleach of all clothing and bedding of smallpox patients, are mandatory. Surface decontamination** is best achieved by using **5% hypochlorite** or **quaternary ammonia** solutions for all exposed surfaces.

TOXINS

BOTULINUM TOXIN

Clostridial neurotoxins (seven related types, classified as A to G) are arguably the most potent toxic substances known to man. Most relevant as the agents causing disease in humans are toxins produced by *Clostridium botulinum*, *C. butyricum*, and *C. barati*. All of these Gram-positive, spore-forming anaerobic bacteria are found in soils and marine sediments throughout the world. In addition, *C. botulinum* can be found in household dust, on the surfaces of foods, and even in honey, whose ingestion is considered a strong risk factor for the disease. Infection with *C. botulinum* results in three epidemiologic forms of botulism:

- Food-borne
- Infantile
- Wound

Botulinum toxin poisoning due to food ingestion is comparatively rare (~1000 annual cases worldwide; ~30 cases in the U.S.). The same is true for the other forms of disease. For this reason, population-wide immunization is not considered practical. As a result, the largely unprotected population constitutes an attractive target for a bioterrorist assault based on the use of botulinum toxins as weapons. The possibility of such use is enhanced by the ease of large-scale production (e.g., in the process of industrial fermentation) and the ease of dissemination (either as aerosols or as direct contaminants of food and water). Paradoxically, botulinum toxins are routinely used to treat spastic disorders and in cosmetology as wrinkle-removing agents.

The history of botulism as a biological weapon dates to World War II. It is possible that Reinhard Heydrich, the infamous Deputy Reichsprotektor of Bohemia and Moravia, was assassinated by British-trained members of Czech resistance using a British-manufactured hand grenade containing both standard explosives and botulinum bacteria. Several terrorist groups have effectively weaponized botulinum and Iraq deployed but did not use munitions containing this toxin. The alluring nature of botulinum toxin as a terrorist tool is severely mitigated by the fact that due to its limited operational efficacy it can be used only against highly specific targets:

- **Normal environmental conditions denature the toxin within ≤12 hours**
- **Sunshine exposure destroys botulinum toxins in 1 to 3 hours**
- **Heat produces denaturation in 1 to 30 minutes; the speed of deactivation increases rapidly at temperatures ≥85°C**
- Approximately 20 minutes of exposure to 3 mg/l or 0.4% free active chlorine (FAC), i.e., concentrations similar to those used in disinfection and municipal water treatment, is sufficient to degrade botulinum toxin by nearly 100%

Mode of Action

Botulinum-type toxins inhibit the release of acetylcholine neurotransmitters at both nicotinic (motor) and muscarinic (cholinergic autonomic) receptors, resulting in deficiencies of neurotransmitters at the synapses (presynaptic inhibition).

CONTRARY TO TREATMENT OF POISONING WITH NERVE GASES AND OTHER AGENTS THAT ACT AT CHOLINERGIC NERVE ENDINGS, ATROPINE SHOULD NEVER BE USED TO TREAT BOTULISM BECAUSE IT MAY AGGRAVATE SYMPTOMS.

Inhalational Botulism

- No cases of inhalational botulism have been described. However, aerosolization of the toxin is possible and has been described
- Symptoms of inhalational botulism are similar to those of the food-borne form
- Neurological symptoms occur 24 to 72 hours after exposure

Food-Borne Botulism

Signs and Symptoms

- Onset between 12 and 48 hours, depending on severity of exposure; may be shorter if triggered by a biological warfare or terrorism event
- Low-dose exposures in primates lead to substantial delays in symptomatology
- Patients are **afebrile and responsive ("feeling like catching a cold")**
- Normal or bradycardiac heart rate with normotension **(CHARACTERISTIC SIGN)**
- Postural hypotension

- Dry mouth and sore throat
- Possibility of dry and encrusted mucosal membranes
- Ileus, constipation, and urinary retention
- Nausea, vomiting, and diarrhea **PRECEDE** neurological symptoms
- Constipation **FOLLOWS** appearance of neurological symptoms
- Variable degrees of skeletal muscle weakness

Clinical Features

- Symmetric neurological symptomatology **(CHARACTERISTIC SIGN)**
- Prominence of cranial nerve palsies **(EARLY CHARACTERISTIC SIGN)**
- Only sensory deficit is blurred vision due to ophthalmoplegia, mydriasis (extreme pupil dilatation), diplopia, ptosis, photophobia
- Dysphonia
- Dysphagia
- Dysarthria
- Symmetrical, descending, and progressive flaccid muscle paralysis extending from neck to arms and legs is a **CHARACTERISTIC NEUROLOGICAL SYMPTOM** of botulinum intoxication
- Possible respiratory failure due to the collapse of weak oropharyngeal musculature

Infantile Botulism

Signs and Symptoms

- Incubation period: 3 to 30 days
- Constipation (≥3 days without defecation)
- Listlessness
- Lethargy
- Weak cry
- Difficulty in sucking and swallowing
- Generalized muscle weakness and hypotonia characterized by poor head control and "frog leg" sign

Clinical Features

- Ptosis
- Ophthalmoplegia
- Slow pupillary light response

- Facial flaccidity
- Dysphagia
- Weak gag reflex
- Poor anal sphincter tone

Wound Botulism

Signs and Symptoms

- Incubation period: typically 10 days
- Symptomatology similar to that of **food-borne** botulism
- Gastrointestinal manifestations are **absent**
- Fever only if wound infection by bacteria other than *Clostridium* is also present

Differential Diagnosis

- Diphtheria
- Congenital neuropathy or myopathy
- Encephalitis
- Guillain–Barré syndrome
- Hypermagnesemia
- Myasthenia gravis
- Mushroom poisoning
- Tick paralysis

Laboratory Tests

General

- **Before** treatment with antiserum, obtain 10 to 15 ml serum, 25 to 50 g feces, 25 to 50 ml gastric fluid, and (if possible) samples of the contaminated food
- **Refrigerate** samples before sending for analysis
- Mouse bioassay for toxin presence
- Mouse toxin neutralization test for toxin identification
- Bedside electromyogram is a rapid method for confirming clinical diagnosis; the trace shows a pattern of numerous, brief, low-amplitude motor unit potentials
- Polymerase chain reaction methods are still experimental

Food-Borne Botulism

- Toxin in serum in ~40% of cases

- Toxin in stool in ~24% of cases
- Clostridia in stool in ~55% of cases
- Stool cultures more sensitive than serum samples during later stages (>3 days)

Infantile Botulism

- Stool and enema fluid are specimens of choice
- Serum is rarely positive

Wound Botulism

- Serum or wound specimen culture best for toxin detection

Treatment

- **DO NOT USE ATROPINE; IT EXACERBATES SYMPTOMS!**
- No specific drug treatment available
- Early administration of trivalent equine botulinum antitoxin is essential as soon diagnosis is made: one vial (10 ml) of antitoxin IV for adult and pediatric administration
- Use of equine antitoxin requires skin testing for horse serum sensitivity
- Supportive care essential; endotracheal intubation or tracheostomy may be a lifesaving step
- **Infant botulism**: complete respiratory failure is typical; intubation is mandatory and may be required for 16 to 23 days; tracheostomy not required
- Monitor respiration (spirometry), peripheral oxygenation of blood (pulse oximetry), and arterial blood gases
- Mechanical ventilation essential when absolute or relative hypercarbia and rapidly progressing hypoxemia are observed; subsequent ventilator support may be needed for several weeks
- **Food-borne botulism:** enemas and cathartics may be used in the absence of ileus to remove the toxin from the intestines; emetics and gastric lavage may also be used if ingestion of contaminated food took place within a few hours of presentation
- **Wound botulism:** thorough debridement of the wound site is mandatory regardless of wound appearance (e.g., even if it looks as if it is healing well)
  - *Create aerobic conditions either by injecting 3% hydrogen peroxide into the wound or flush it with hyperbaric oxygen*
  - *Urinary catheter may be needed if urine retention is present*

Prophylaxis

- Experimental pentavalent toxoid of *C. botulinum* toxin A,B,C, and D types is available but its efficacy is unknown despite administration to several thousand volunteers and high-risk personnel; serum antitoxin levels produced in humans correspond to protective levels exhibited in animal studies
- Administer vaccine to individuals and groups who have potential for botulinum toxin aerosol exposure (e.g., laboratory personnel)
- Postexposure vaccination data from animal models are available; no human data exist

Precautionary Measures

Botulism is **noncontagious**. Under normal circumstances, it can be easily prevented by implementation of most standard, common-sense sanitary precautions — washing hands, cleaning fruits and vegetables in hot water, avoiding spoiled canned and prepared foods, etc. Since clostridia are very sensitive to atmosphere, sunshine, temperature, and standard decontamination agents, standard hospital precautions and disinfection measures are fully adequate during emergency treatment and ensuing hospital recovery even in the event of a bioterrorist attack that affects large numbers of people. Remember:

- **Normal environmental conditions denature the toxin within ≤12 hours**
- **Sunshine exposure destroys botulinum toxins in 1 to 3 hours**
- **Heat produces denaturation in 1 to 30 minutes; the speed of deactivation increases rapidly at temperatures ≥85°C.**
- Approximately 20 minutes exposure to 3 mg/l or 0.4% free active chlorine (FAC) in concentrations similar to those used in disinfection and municipal water treatment procedures is sufficient to degrade botulinum toxin by nearly 100%

The major impact of a botulinum toxin-based terrorist attack would be psychological, and its consequences may be devastating. Unfortunately, as most other biological weapons, no effective means of early detection of botulinum toxin exist. The first indicator of large-scale exposure would probably be the hospital arrival of several victims with signs of botulism.

Replacing the present lack of awareness on the part of the general public with the knowledge about early recognition of botulinum symptoms could significantly increase chances of recovery making the difference between widespread panic and a relatively well contained incident. Prevention of such panic reaction can be achieved only through an immediate, fact-based awareness campaign directed by the public health authorities and utilizing all accessible media.

RICIN TOXIN

Ricin is a powerful toxin derived from the castor plant, *Ricinus communics*. The toxic effects of ricin were recognized in ancient times. While its potency does not match bacterial or viral biological warfare agents, its potential for such applications rests in the ease and low cost of manufacture and stability in liquid, crystalline, lyophilized, and aerosolized forms.

Although ricin oil manufacture ceased in the U.S., nearly 1 million tons of castor beans are processed for oil worldwide. The toxin remains in the waste mash and can be extracted via a simple chemical process. Because it is readily available, ricin found lethal application during the Cold War when the Bulgarian intelligence service Drazven Sigurnost and the Soviet KGB assassinated Georgi Markov, a Bulgarian dissident living in London, in 1978. Several other cases of the use of ricin as an assassination weapon were reported in the late 1970s and early 1980s. In the U.S., attempts to employ ricin as a bioterrorist weapon or as an instrument of murder led to convictions of the implicated individuals.

Although highly popularized by the press, ricin is not an effective biological weapon. Its toxicity, while high, is nearly 1000-fold less than that of botulinum and a very large amount would be required to produce the effects expected of an effective biological warfare agent. Its potential as a destabilizing agent and as a weapon against specific targets remains high because of its ready availability and multiple dissemination modes. Aerosol exposure, injection, or ingestion as food or drink may all lead to a lethal outcome.

Mode of Action

Ricin is potent cytotoxin whose toxicity appears to vary with the route of administration and amount absorbed. However, once inside a cell, a single ricin molecule can deactivate over 1500 ribosomes/minute, leading to rapid cell death. After release into the cytosol, ricin's A chain (ricin consists of A and B polypeptide chains and two hemagglutinins) acts as a potent inhibitor of DNA replication and protein synthesis. Recognition of these properties served as the basis for experimental attempts to use ricin as a tumor growth inhibitor.

Signs and Symptoms

Inhalation

- **Initial symptoms** (within 4 to 8 hours postexposure):
  - *Weakness*
  - *Acute onset of fever*

- *Cough*
- *Dyspnea*
- *Nausea and vomiting*
- *Chest tightness*
- *Arthralgia*
■ **Delayed symptoms** (8 to 18 hours postexposure):
  - *Sweating*
  - *Cough*
  - *Dyspnea*
  - *Pulmonary edema*
  - *Cyanosis*
■ **Late symptoms** (18 to 24 hours postexposure):
  - *Airway necrosis (suppurative lesions)*
  - *Pulmonary edema due to pulmonary capillary leak*
  - *Rhinitis*
  - *Laryngitis*
  - *Hypotension*
■ Respiratory and cardiovascular collapse within 36 to 72 hours of exposure

Injection

■ Very rapid onset of symptoms (<4 hours)
■ **Small doses** (<20 µg) produce flu-like symptoms, fatigue (may be severe), myalgia, nausea, and vomiting
■ **Large doses** (>200 µg) produce:
  - *General symptoms similar to those from inhalation exposure*
  - *Muscle and lymph node necrosis surrounding the injection site.*
  - *Significantly elevated white blood count*
  - *Possible hypotension and tachycardia at late stages*
  - *Gastrointestinal hemorrhage*
  - *Liver necrosis*
  - *Diffuse nephritis*
  - *Diffuse splenitis*
  - *Mild pulmonary perivascular edema*

Ingestion

■ Very rapid onset of symptoms (<4 hours)
■ Mild pulmonary perivascular edema
■ Vomiting

- Abdominal pain
- Hematemesis
- Diarrhea (may be bloody)
- Anuria
- Vascular collapse and death within 3 to 4 days

Clinical Features

- Rapid definitive diagnosis is **extremely difficult in isolated cases** (e.g., assassination by injection)
- Diagnosis in cases of food and water contamination is based on a **combination of clinical and epidemiological features:**
  - *Clinical presentation of a large number of patients with symptoms of* **acute lung injury**, *all coming from the same area; possibility of aerosol exposure*
  - *Clinical presentation of a large number of patients with symptoms of* **severe gastroenteritis or hemorrhagic gastroenteritis**, *all coming from the same area; possibility of food or water contamination*
- Differential diagnosis **must** consider other biological and chemical warfare threats that present similar symptomatologies, i.e., **SEB, Q fever, tularemia, plague, and poisoning from chemical agents such as phosgene**
- Ricin-induced pulmonary edema starts much later (1 to 3 days postexposure) than that induced by SEB (~12 hours postexposure) and phosgene (6 hours postexposure)
- Unlike SEB, ricin poisoning produces no clinical plateau
- Unlike infectious processes, ricin intoxication progresses despite antibiotic treatment
- Ricin intoxication is not associated with the widened mediastinum seen in anthrax

Differential Diagnosis

- Anthrax
- Cholera
- Phosgene (and other lung damaging chemical warfare agents)
- Plague
- Q fever
- Salmonella poisoning
- SEB poisoning

Laboratory Tests

- Complete blood count: **neutrophilic leukocytosis**
- Other routine laboratory tests are typically nonspecific
- Chest x-ray may reveal infiltrates or acute respiratory distress syndrome
- ELISA, ECL, and immunocytochemistry for toxin detection and definitive diagnosis
- Sequential specimen sampling:
  - *0 to 24 hours postexposure: nasal swabs, induced respirator secretions for ELISA and/or PCR, serum for toxin assay*
  - *24 to 36 hours postexposure: serum for toxin assay, tissue for immunohistochemistry*
  - *>6 days: serum for IgM and IgG*

Treatment

- **NO DEFINITIVE TREATMENT EXISTS**
- Suggested approaches depend on the route of exposure but are only supportive

Inhalation

- Oxygen
  - *Intubation*
  - *Ventilation*
  - *PEEP*
  - *Hemodynamic monitoring*
  - *Treat pulmonary edema if needed*
  - *Anti-inflammatory and/or analgesic agents may be considered*

Ingestion

- Gastric lavage
- Cathartics (e.g., magnesium citrate)
- Activated charcoal has limited value against molecules as large as ricin
- Fluid replacement

Injection

- Rapid removal of the foreign body causing release of the toxin is essential

- Depending on disease stage, subsequent treatment should be similar to treatment for inhalation and ingestion exposure
- Update tetanus vaccination status if unknown
- Antibiotics may be considered to prevent secondary infection, e.g., 1 to 2 g cefazolin IV/IM q 6 to 8 hours

Prophylaxis

- All active immunization and passive prophylaxis measures are experimental; promising data are based on animal studies only
- In experimental studies, postexposure administration of specific antibodies proved ineffective in preventing ricin-induced pathological effects

Precautionary Measures

Although ricin poisoning cannot be transferred from person to person and ricin cannot be passed through secondary aerosolization, standard precautions and decontamination measures are mandatory. A protective mask serves as a sufficient barrier even in the presence of an aerosol attack. The risk of secondary dermal absorption during rescue operations is small, and soap and water decontamination of exposed skin is sufficient to eliminate that risk entirely.

Patient decontamination: remove clothing and wash with soap and water. Further decontamination with 0.5% sodium hypochlorite solution may be conducted. Do not use the solution on the eyes or open abdominal, cranial, or spinal cord injuries. The solution can be used to decontaminate superficial, noncavity wounds. Suction into disposable containers: the toxin is deactivated and nonhazardous within 5 minutes. Ricin is also deactivated by heat (10 minutes at $\geq 80°C$ or 60 minutes at $\geq 50°C$). Low concentrations of chlorine (≤ 10 mg/l free active chlorine) or iodine (≤ 16 mg/l) exert no effects on ricin.

STAPHYLOCOCCAL ENTEROTOXIN B (SEB)

SEB and six other enterotoxins produced by *Staphylococcus aureus* strains belong to a group of so-called superantigens capable of inducing devastating pathophysiological effects due to their very high potencies as activators of the immune system. It is believed that cytokines resulting from the activation of the immune system are the primary mediators of the toxic effects of SEB.

Staphylococci are among common pathogens that thrive on unrefrigerated meats, dairy, and bakery products. Under typical circumstances, the toxin excreted by the bacteria (exotoxin) induces its intestinal effects after ingestion of contaminated food. The resultant poisoning, while nonlethal, is severely incapacitating and the illness lasts as long as 2 weeks.

SEB has been extensively studied as a potential biological warfare agent. It can be aerosolized, it is stable, and it can induce considerable systemic damage including multiorgan failure, shock-like syndrome, and even death, particularly after high concentration exposures. Nonetheless, the consequences of SEB administered at even very low doses can be devastating. Some authors indicate that aerosol dispersion of SEB on a battlefield may produce up to 80% incapacitation. As a result of bioterrorism action, the numbers of affected populations would be significantly lower. In both cases, the major impact would arise from the incapacitating properties of the toxin rather than its lethality. Due to the duration of the illness, many daily activities within the affected community would be disrupted or cease entirely. A widespread panic reaction enhancing social destabilization would be a further consequence of a terrorist assault using SEB.

Mechanism of Action

The toxin binds to Type II receptors of the major histocompatibility complex (MHC). The binding stimulates T cells and leads to their rapid proliferation. Systemic effects of the toxin are thought to result from massive release of γ-interferon (γINF), interleukins 1,2, and 6 (IL1,2,6), and α-tumor necrosis factor (αTNF) from mast cells. Intense inflammatory reaction follows, resulting in tissue injury of the host. Clinical features of intoxication are specific for the mode of exposure (inhalation vs. ingestion) but morbidity is significant in both cases.

Signs and Symptoms

- Physical examination typically unremarkable
- Postural weakness due to fluid loss following ingestion may be present

- Occasional conjunctivitis
- Chest x-ray normal except when pulmonary edema develops (see section on inhalation poisoning)

Ingestion (Food Poisoning)

- Follows swallowing of improperly refrigerated, stored, or handled foodstuffs
- Onset 3 to 12 hours after ingestion
- Acute salivation
- Nausea
- Vomiting
- Abdominal cramps
- Diarrhea
- Possibility of fluid loss
- High exposure doses may induce septic shock and death
- Most cases are self-limiting and resolve within ≤24 hours

Inhalation

- Onset 3 to 12 hours after exposure
- Fever of 39.5 to 41°C (103 to 106°F) may last 2 to 5 days
- Prostration
- Chills
- Headache
- Myalgia
- Nonproductive cough
- In severe cases:
  - *Dyspnea and retrosternal chest pain*
  - *No evidence of consolidations or effusions*
  - *Reflective tachycardia*
  - *Gastrointestinal symptoms* **possible** *due to inadvertent secondary ingestion of toxin*
- In very severe cases:
  - *Frank pulmonary edema due to capillary leak*
  - *Possibility of acute respiratory distress syndrome (ARDS)*

Clinical Features

- Diagnosis, especially of inhalational exposure, based on a combination of clinical and epidemiological features. Be prepared for unclear initial diagnosis. Keep in mind that:

- *Cases of natural influenza and pneumonia present over longer periods*
- *Staphylococcus-induced food poisoning presents without pulmonary symptoms*
- *SEB intoxication produces a rapid clinical plateau, followed by stabilization*

■ Inhalational anthrax, tularemia, and pneumonic plague progress when untreated; SEB does not
■ No infiltrates present on chest x-ray with SEB; infiltrates appear with tularemia, plague, and Q fever
■ No neurological findings with SEB; botulism and nerve agents present neurological findings
■ Early respiratory difficulties with SEB; late difficulties with botulism
■ SEB attack will result in large number of patients presenting within a 24-hour period; laboratory findings are unhelpful:
  - *Possible nonspecific elevation of neutrophilic leukocytes and elevated thrombocyte sedimentation rate*
  - *Toxin identifiable in nasal swabs for 12 to 24 hours following exposure to inhalational SEB*

Differential Diagnosis

■ ARDS
■ Bowel obstruction
■ Cholecystitis
■ Gastritis
■ Gastroenteritis
■ Hypovolemic shock
■ Lung-damaging chemical warfare agents
■ Nerve agents
■ Pancreatitis
■ Pericarditis
■ Ricin
■ Scorpion envenomation

Laboratory Tests

■ Laboratory findings unhelpful
■ ELISA, polymerase chain reaction
■ Serum sampling as early as possible; toxin may be difficult to detect
■ Urine samples – SEB toxin may be detected easily

- Acute and convalescent serum samples may help definitive diagnosis retrospectively; data will be important for public health authorities
- Chest x-ray will show pulmonary edema and ARDS only following aerosol exposure (only in severe cases)

Treatment

- Limited to supportive care
- Vigorous fluid replacement
- Humidified oxygen in patients with inhalational SEB
- Acetaminophen and cough suppressants for general comfort; the value of steroids is uncertain
- In severe cases with evident pulmonary edema and ARDS, proceed with intubation, mechanical ventilation, diuretics (furosemide, 40 mg IV), and vasopressors:
  - *Dopamine (5 to 20 µg/kg, titrate until patient responds)*
  - *Norepinephrine if blood pressure remains <70 mmHg (8 to 12 µg/minute loading dose followed by 2 to 4 µg/minute IV infusion)*

Prophylaxis

- No vaccine available
- Primates protected by experimental immunization

Precautionary Measures

Standard precautions: toxin is deactivated after heating ~5 minutes at 100°C. Surface decontamination with 0.5% sodium hypochlorite for 10 to 15 minutes and/or use large amounts of soap and water.

SAXITOXIN

In 1987, marine biologists noticed large numbers of deaths among hump-back whales. The mortality approached the cumulative number of dead animals during the previous 50 years. Later the same year, following two more such incidents in Canada and Guatemala, nearly 30 persons were dead and several hundred incapacitated by a severely incapacitating disease. Eventually, the illness was associated with the ingestion of contaminated mollusks with dinoflagellate algae of predominantly *Gon-yalux* species.

The 20 shellfish toxins whose ingestion results in **paralytic shellfish poisoning (PSP)** are all derivatives of saxitoxin. While ingestion of all shellfish poses the risk of intoxication, PSP is typically associated with mussels, clams, cockles, and scallops. The toxins are very potent. The symptomatology produced by intoxication leads frequently to misdiagnosis and underreporting. Like other biotoxins, saxitoxin has many uses in pharmacological research. However, since saxitoxin is approximately 1000 times more potent than paralyzing warfare agents such sarin, it has a great interest among groups that advocate chemical and biological warfare. In 1970, President Nixon ordered the Central Intelligence Agency to destroy its entire stock of the compound within 5 years. Congressional hearings revealed that the agency retained approximately 10 g.

Although saxitoxin can be isolated from contaminated mollusks or manufactured as a synthetic product, its applications as a large-scale bioterrorist weapon are limited. Production is difficult and requires significant knowledge and complex equipment. Moreover, since saxitoxin is among Schedule 1 agents cited by the Chemical Weapons Convention its distribution, even for research purposes, is under strict control. The most likely bioterrorist use of saxitoxin would be target-specific and predominantly for assassination. Aerosolization and limited contamination are remote possibilities.

Mode of Action

Saxitoxin is a water soluble, potent, selective, and reversible antagonist (blocker) of voltage-dependent sodium channels that does not affect the fluxes of other ions (chloride, potassium, calcium) or neurotransmitter release. Physiologically, the effect of saxitoxin manifests most strikingly as the blockade of nerve impulses (conduction block) in motor neurons and muscles.

Signs and Symptoms

No data on inhalational effects of saxitoxin in humans are available. Animal studies indicate compression of symptoms listed below and death as early as minutes after exposure. The effects of projectile injection of saxitoxin are unknown.

The following symptoms of ingestion appear rapidly, sometimes as soon as 5 to 30 minutes after ingestion:

- Early symptoms:
  - *Tingling of lips, tongue, and fingertips (**CHARACTERISTIC SIGN**)*
  - *Aphasia*
  - *Salivation*
  - *Intense thirst*
  - *Headache*
- Numbness of neck and extremities within 4 to 6 hours (**CHARACTERISTIC SIGN**)
- Ataxia and general weakness
- Sensation of floating in air
- Induced reflexes and consciousness are intact
- Involvement of cranial nerves
- Less frequent signs: nausea, vomiting, diarrhea, and abdominal pain
- Severe poisoning:
  - *Progressively worsening respiratory distress*
  - *Flaccid muscular paralysis within 2 to 12 hours postingestion*
  - *Death due to respiratory collapse within 2 to 12 hours*

Clinical Features

- Laboratory findings nonspecific; elevation of serum creatine kinase reported in some cases
- Cardiac arrhythmias possible
- Mild hypotension
- **Ciguatera toxins** characterized by prominence of gastrointestinal manifestations
- **Tetradotoxin** induces significant hypotension; tetradotoxin poisoning **only** after eating fish
- Dehydration
- Definitive diagnosis based on ELISA and high performance liquid chromatography (HPLC)
- Mouse test recommended as standard toxin identification measure

Differential Diagnosis

- Carbamate
- Ciguatera toxin
- Gastroenteritis
- Organophosphate
- Phenytoin
- Tetradotoxin

Laboratory Tests

- Serum tests unavailable
- ELISA, HPLC, and mouse bioassay are time consuming or require specialized equipment

Treatment

- Supportive and symptom-driven
- Aggressive respiratory support up to mechanical ventilation essential at any sign of respiratory compromise
- Aggressive fluid replacement
- Diuresis may enhance toxin elimination
- Gastrointestinal decontamination with activated charcoal may be performed; its value is uncertain
- Activated charcoal, 1 g/kg PO (with or without cathartic)
- **Neostygmine** (0.5 to 2 mg **IV**) and **edrophonium** (2 to 10 mg/kg) have been used as countermeasures to treat muscle weakness in **tetradotoxin** intoxication **(the effects of these drugs for saxitoxin poisoning are unknown)**

Prophylaxis

No prophylactic measure is effective in the context of bioterrorism activity. Under other circumstances, avoidance of consumption of shellfish harvested outside regularly surveyed areas or harvested during periods associated with dinoflagellate blooms (red tides) is the only effective step. Antitoxin therapy has been successfully tested in animals but clinical efficacy studies have not been performed. No vaccine against saxitoxin has been developed.

Precautionary Measures

Saxitoxin poisoning poses no risk of transmission from person to person. However, even if no reports of secondary inhalational exposure exist, the very high toxicity of the substance combined with minute amounts required to induce poisoning (0.2 mg is fatal for an average human) makes maintenance of standard precautions advisable. Routine decontamination measures (0.5% hypochlorite solution, 16 mg/l iodine, and even thorough soap and water cleanup) offer sufficient means to deactivate saxitoxin. Due to its heat resistance only a prolonged (>20 minutes) exposure to >>100°C will lead to sufficient deactivation.

T2 (TRICHOTHECENE) TOXINS

Mycotoxins belong to a large group (more than 40) of highly toxic compounds produced by a variety of molds. Trichothecene toxins are synthesized by a number of species belonging to genera *Trichoderma, Fusarium, Cephalosporium, Myrotecium, Verticimonosporium,* and *Stachybotrys. Fusarium* fungi grow readily on barley, corn, oats, rye, and wheat. During World War II, consumption of bread baked from *Fusarium*-contaminated wheat flour resulted in the deaths of thousands of Russian civilians — an event that focused attention on the chemistry and biological effects of trichothecenes.

T2 toxins are attractive warfare agents. Their potent toxic effects can be attained through a variety of entry routes. Transdermal, inhalational, and ingestion exposures produce symptoms of intoxication. In biological warfare, T2 toxins would be dispersed as aerosols. Numerous reports alleged use of trichoecene toxins during the conflicts in Vietnam, Laos, Kampuchea, and Afghanistan. There are indications that T2 agents were used also against Yemeni royalists, and as components of chemical and biological weapons during the war between Iran and Iraq. Conservative estimates suggest that at least 10,000 people, chiefly civilians, died from attacks with munitions containing T2 toxins or as a result of their aerial dispersal.

Yellow rain is the popular name for aerosol dispersal of T2 toxins, and derives from the sound of sticky, yellow liquid landing on foliage during the conflict in Laos. Other accounts mention yellow clouds of mist or smoke or insecticide-like spray. Brown, red, green, or white mists or vapors have also been associated with alleged T2 attacks. Controversy surrounds the reality of T2 toxin battlefield use during the Southeast Asian conflicts. Nonetheless, the potential for antipersonnel use of trichothecene toxins is real enough to be a source of concern. The use of T2 compounds for bioterrorism is more problematic due to comparatively large amounts of the toxin needed to be effective. Hence, an assault involving T2 agents would have to be targeted selectively rather than used on large groups to produce numerous casualties.

T2 toxins are extremely stable and resist inactivation by heat and ultraviolet light. A brief exposure to sodium hypochlorite destroys the compounds. However, their stability and ease of storage in aerosol form make them particularly suitable for aerial dusting of crops by bioterrorists. This method of T2 toxin dispersion must be borne in mind when large numbers of casualties present with symptoms of intense skin irritation.

The onset of symptoms is extremely rapid (MINUTES after the exposure). At lower concentrations such as would be expected following aerial spraying of crops, T2 toxins can be considered primarily as very potent skin and eye irritants. However, large concentrations can produce incapacitation and death within hours or even minutes. Importantly, while many symptoms resulting from T2 exposure are similar to those induced by chemical vesicants (mustard gas), chemical vesicants have **characteristic odors. T2 toxin exposure will produce no olfactory effects.**

Mode of Action

The exact mechanisms involved in T2 toxicity are unclear, but involve potent inhibition of nucleic acid and protein synthesis, reduced efficiency of mitochondrial respiration, and alterations of cell membrane structures and functions. All these effects are particularly prominent in rapidly dividing cells (bone marrow, mucosal epithelium of the GI tract, skin, etc.) and result in effects that closely mimic radiation sickness. For this reason T2 toxins are also known as "radiomimetic" substances.

Signs and Symptoms

Typical Symptom Complex

- Burning skin pain
- Blistering
- Redness
- Pruritus
- Rash and blisters
- Dyspnea
- Vomiting
- Diarrhea

Dermal Exposure

- Symptoms appear within minutes to hours:
  – *Intense burning pain*
  – *Pruritus*
  – *Redness*
  – *Blistering*
  – *Necrosis and sloughing in **lethal cases***

Ocular Exposure

- Symptoms appear within minutes:
  – *Pain*
  – *Redness*

     – *Blurred vision*
     – *Foreign body sensation*

Inhalation Exposure

- Symptoms appear within minutes to hours
- Nose (minutes):
  - *Nasal itching and pain*
  - *Sneezing*
  - *Rhinorrhea*
  - *Epistaxis*
- Mouth and throat (minutes):
  - *Pain*
  - *Hemoptysis*
  - *Ulcerative pharyngitis*
- Tracheobronchial and pulmonary (minutes):
  - *Dyspnea*
  - *Wheezing*
  - *Cough*

Ingestion Exposure

- Symptoms appear within minutes to <2 hours
- Anorexia
- Nausea
- Vomiting
- Abdominal cramps
- Bloody diarrhea
- Systemic symptoms (hours):
  - *Prostration*
  - *Weakness*
  - *Ataxia*
  - *Collapse*

Severe/Fatal Cases

- Hypothermia
- Tachycardia
- Hypotension
- Shock

■ Death occurs within hours or even days; may occur within minutes in particularly severe cases

Clinical Features

■ Combination of clinical and epidemiological factors provides significant indicators:
- *Large number of victims with characteristic symptomatology*
- *Large number of dead animals of a variety of species*
- *Physical evidence of pigmented oily liquids*
■ T2 toxins are odorless and symptoms are immediate. Mustard gas and other vesicant agents are visible, have odors, and produce delayed symptoms
■ T2 toxins involve skin; SEB and ricin exposures include no skin components

Differential Diagnosis

■ Radiation sickness
■ Ricin
■ SEB
■ Vesicant (blistering) warfare agents

Laboratory Tests

■ No diagnostic kit is available
■ Pronounced but transient leukocytosis
■ Reduced hematocrit
■ Serum proteins unaffected
■ Gas chromatography and HPLC for definitive detection of T2 toxins in plasma and urine
■ Urine is the sampling fluid of choice. Add 0.1 ml concentrated HCl per 100 ml urine (no need for refrigeration)

Treatment

■ No antidote is available
■ All treatment is supportive
■ All patient clothing should be removed
■ Irrigate eyes with copious amounts of saline or uncontaminated water.
■ Thoroughly wash the skin with soap and uncontaminated water **even if treatment is delayed by <6 hours**

- Use **calamine** or **0.25% camphor and methanol** to relieve dermal irritation
- Skin decontamination kits available **only to military personnel**
- Respiratory support may be required
- Steam inhalation and/or cough suppressants (e.g., codeine) in mild cases of inhalatory exposure
- Standard burn support for extensive dermal exposure
- Standard poison therapy **including activated charcoal** for ingestion **Superactivated charcoal** may be more effective
- **Dexamethasone (1 to 10 mg/kg IV) in animal studies administered <3 hours postexposure improved survival and reduced bloody diarrhea**
- **Benedryl** (diphenhydramine) and **naloxone** administered before and after T2 exposure prolonged survival when given topically or SQ to **mice**

Prophylaxis

- No prophylactic measures are available
- Immunological (monoclonal antibodies) and chemical protectants have been studied but are not available
- Ascorbic acid (400 to 1200 mg/kg IP) reduced lethality **in animals**. No human data available

Precautionary Measures

T2 toxins are extremely stable and neither autoclaving nor ultraviolet light reduces their bioactivities. Exposure to 1500°F for 30 minutes will lead to inactivation. Environmental decontamination with **hypochlorite solution is not effective** although addition of 0.1 M NaOH to 1% hypochlorite and exposure of the contaminated surface for 1 hour will result in inactivation.

Standard precautions for healthcare personnel are mandatory. Since clothing items of human victims of T2 exposure will serve as toxin reservoirs, all outer garments must be removed. Patients should be washed thoroughly with **soap and water within 4 hours following exposure.** The removed clothing must be decontaminated by **soaking for 6 to 10 hours in 5% hypochlorite solution**.

4

PEDIATRIC TREATMENT

BACTERIAL DISEASES

ANTHRAX

Immediate Treatment

- Ciprofloxacin 20 to 30 mg/kg IV q 12 hours (not to exceed 1.0 qd); **ORAL ADMINISTRATION IS INEFFECTIVE**
- Penicillin G 100,000 to 150,000 U/kg/d IV divided q 4 to 6 hours

Maintenance Treatment

- Ciprofloxacin 15 mg/kg PO q 12 hours, 60 days or 10 mg/kg IV q 12 hours, 60 days (not to exceed 400 mg/dose)
- Doxycycline <45 kg body weight: 2.2 mg/kg PO or IV q 12 hours, 60 days; >45 kg body weight: same dose as adult

BRUCELLOSIS

- Oral antibiotics: consult an infectious disease specialist for a definitive regimen
- Regimens of choice:
  - *Doxycycline 5 mg/kg qd PO 21 days plus rifampin 10 to 20 mg/kg qd IV 21 days (rifampin not to exceed 600 mg qd)*
  - *Doxycycline 5 mg/kg qd PO 21 days plus streptomycin 20 to 40 mg/kg qd IM 21 days (streptomycin not to exceed 1 g qd)*

CHOLERA

■ In suspected cases (prior to definitive diagnosis):

1. Assess dehydration
2. Rehydrate under frequent monitoring
3. Maintain hydration; replace fluid loss until diarrhea stops
4. Administer antibiotic (see below)
5. Feed

■ Tetracycline:
  – *Single dose: 25 mg/kg PO (not to exceed 1 g)*
  – *Multiple dose: 40 mg/kg/d PO divided qid for 3 days (not to exceed 2 g/day)*
■ Doxycycline:
  – *Single dose: 7 mg/kg PO (not to exceed 300 mg)*
  – *Multiple dose: 2 mg/kg PO qd on days 2 and 3 (not to exceed 100 mg/dose)*
■ Ciprofloxacin:
  – *NOT approved*
  – *Single dose: 30 mg/kg PO (not to exceed 1 g)*
  – *Multiple dose: 30 mg/kg/d PO divided qid for 3 days (not to exceed 2 g/day)*
■ In severe cases:
  – *Start IV line with Ringer's lactate solution immediately; if not available, use normal saline*
  – *Patient >1 year old: 30 ml/kg within 30 minutes, then 70 ml/kg in the next 2 hours*
  – *Patient <1 year old: 30 ml/kg within 30 minutes, then 70 ml/kg in the next 5 hours*
  – *Monitor frequently; after initial 30 ml/kg, pulse should be strong and blood pressure normal. If not, continue IV fluid*
  – *Administer ORS solution (5 ml/kg) as soon the patient can drink.*
  – *Reassess infants 6 hours after start of rehydration*
  – *If signs of dehydration persist, maintain hydration using standard guidelines*

For rehydration tables, see **http://www.emedicine.com/ ped/topic382.htm** (Thaker, V.V., Cholera, in *e-Medicine Journal*).

GLANDERS AND MELIOIDOSIS

Treatment varies, depending on the type and severity of the disease.

Localized Form/Mild Toxicity

- Amoxicillin and clavunalate 60 mg/kg qd PO divided tid
- Tetracycline not recommended for children <8 years; 40 mg/kg/d PO divided tid for children >8 years
- TMP/SMX not recommended for infants <2 months; TMP 4 mg/kg qd; SMX 20 mg/kg qd PO divided bid for infants >2 months
- A combination of two regimens is recommended for the initial 30 days followed by monotherapy with either amoxicillin/clavunalate or TMP/sulfa for the next 60 to 150 days

Severe Disease

- Parenteral ceftazidime plus TMP/SMX for 14 days followed by PO therapy for 6 months
- Ceftadizime 25 to 30 mg/kg qd IM divided tid
- TMP/SMX: TMP 4 mg/kg qd; SMX 20 mg/kg qd PO; divided bid
- If plague cannot be ruled out when treatment is initiated, add streptomycin (20 to 40 mg/kg qd IM 21 days; not to exceed 1 g qd)

PLAGUE

- Treatment for 10 to 14 days; patient usually afebrile within 3 to 4 days
- Streptomycin 20 to 40 mg/kg qd IM 7 to 14 days or until patient is afebrile for 5 to 7 days, not to exceed 0.75 to 1 g/day
- Gentamicin dose not established
- Doxycycline:
  - *Not recommended for children <8 years*
  - *For children >8 years, 2 to 5 mg/kg qd in 1 or 2 doses, not to exceed 200 mg/day*
- Chloramphenicol 50 to 75 mg/kg qd IM/IV divided q 6

Q FEVER

Consult an infectious diseases specialist about choices of antibiotics and durations of treatment.

Acute Form

- Tetracycline:
  - *Not recommended for children <8 years*

– For children >8 years, 25 to 50 mg/kg qd PO divided q 6 hours
■ Doxycycline:
  – Not recommended for children <8 years
  – For children >8 years, 2 to 5 mg/kg PO/IV q 12 hours, not to exceed 200 mg/day

Chronic Form

■ Tetracycline or doxycycline (in combination with TMP-SMX)
■ See entries for treating acute Q fever (above) for doses of tetracycline or doxycycline
■ TMP 4 mg/kg qd//SMX 20 mg/kg qd PO; divided bid
■ Rifampin 10 to 20 mg/kg PO/IV, not to exceed 600 mg/d

Tularemia

■ Course of treatment for all drugs: 10 to 14 days
■ Streptomycin considered agent of choice; 20 to 40 mg/kg qd IM 7 to 14 days or until patient is afebrile for 5 to 7 days, not to exceed 0.75 to 1 g/day
■ Tetracycline not recommended for children <8 years
■ For children >8 years, 25 to 50 mg/kg tetracycline qd PO divided q 6 hours
■ Ciprofloxacin 30 mg/kg/day PO divided qid for 7 to 14 days, not to exceed 2 g/day

VIRAL DISEASES

EQUINE ENCEPHALOMYELITIS

- No specific treatment available
- Supportive treatment in patients with uncomplicated disease
- Analgesics to relieve headache and myalgia
- In clinical encephalitis patients, specialist treatment involving anti-convulsants, fluid and electrolyte balance support, and airway maintenance may be required

VIRAL HEMORRHAGIC FEVERS

- Ribavarin: no pediatric dosage established
- Adult dosing is 30 mg/kg IV load followed by 15 mg/kg q 6 hours for 4 days, followed by 7.5 mg/kg q 8 hours for 6 days
- Treatment is most effective if begun within 7 days of onset
- Lower IV doses or 2.0 g PO followed by 1.0 g PO for 10 days may be useful
- Ribavarin treatment is useful for:
  - *Crimean-Congo hemorrhagic fever*
  - *Hanta hemorrhagic fever if started within 4 days of onset.*
  - *Lassa hemorrhagic fever*
  - *Rift Valley hemorrhagic fever*
- Ribavarin is ineffective in treating:
  - *Filoviridae infections (Ebola and Marburg hemorrhagic fevers)*
  - *Flaviviridae infections (Dengue, Kyasanur Forest, and Omsk hemorrhagic fevers and yellow fever)*

SMALLPOX

- No specific treatment available
- Vaccinia immune globulin (VIG) may be of value if given early
- Administer VIG as for adults: 0.6 ml/kg IM
- Hydration to prevent fluid loss caused by fever and breakdown of the skin barrier
- Antibiotics to prevent secondary infection (dosing: see Cholera and Glanders sections)

For rehydration tables, see **http://www.emedicine.com /ped/topic382.htm** (Thaker, V.V., Cholera, in *e-Medicine Journal*).

TOXINS

BOTULINUM TOXIN

- No specific treatment available
- Early administration of trivalent equine botulinum antitoxin essential as soon diagnosis is made
- One vial (10 ml) of antitoxin/adult patient IV once

RICIN TOXIN

- No specific treatment available; suggested approaches depend on route of exposure and are only supportive
- Antibiotics recommended in cases of parenteral (injection) exposure
- Cefazolin 25 to 50 mg/kg/day IV/IM divided q 6 to 8 hours
- If hypotension is present, administer dopamine as for adults:
  - *Low dose: 0.5 to 5 μg/kg/minute IV*
  - *Medium dose: 5 to 10 μg/kg/minute IV*
  - *High dose: >10 μg/kg/minute IV*
- Norepinephrine as for adults: 2 to 4 μg/kg/minute IV; can be increased to 2 to 4 μg/kg/minute q 5 to 10 minutes prn

STAPHYLOCOCCAL ENTEROTOXIN B (SEB)

- If hypotension is present, administer dopamine as for adults:
  - *Low dose: 0.5 to 5 μg/kg/minute IV*
  - *Medium dose: 5 to 10 μg/kg/minute IV*
  - *High dose: >10 μg/kg/minute IV*
- Norepinephrine as for adults: 2 to 4 μg/kg/minute IV; can be increased to 2 to 4 μg/kg/minute q 5 to 10 minutes prn

SAXITOXIN

- Treatment is supportive and symptom-driven
- Aggressive respiratory support up to mechanical ventilation at any sign of respiratory compromise essential
- Aggressive fluid replacement
- Diuresis may enhance toxin elimination

- Gastrointestinal decontamination with activated charcoal may be performed; value is uncertain
  - *Not recommended for children <1 year*
  - *Give 1 g/kg PO with or without cathartic to children >1 year*
- Neostygmine 0.5 to 2 mg/IV
  - *Adult dose used as a countermeasure to muscle weakness in tetradotoxin intoxication in which physiopharmacological features are similar to those of saxitoxin. The effects in saxitoxin poisoning are unknown*
- Edrophonium 2 to 10 mg/kg/IV
  - *Adult dose been used as a countermeasure to muscle weakness in tetradotoxin intoxication in which physiopharmacological features are similar to those of saxitoxin. The effects in saxitoxin poisoning are unknown*

T2 (TRICHOTHECENE) TOXINS

- All treatment is supportive; no antidote is known
- Calamine or 0.25% camphor and methanol to relieve dermal irritation
- Respiratory support may be required
- Steam inhalation and/or cough suppressants (e.g., codeine) in mild cases of inhalatory exposure
- Activated charcoal not recommended for children <1 year
- For children >1 year, 1 g/kg PO with or without cathartic

5

USEFUL PROCEDURES

Many methods and procedures listed below are familiar to experienced healthcare personnel, particularly those working with infectious diseases and emergency medicine. However, many who may face victims of a bioterrorism attack may need a quick reference that will allow them to perform the initial actions required to determine the nature of the presenting illness and the initial treatment of victims.

When time is of the essence and the resources of specialized laboratories are stressed, a room with a sink, power supply, microscope, and a safe receptacle for contaminated material (solid and liquid, including histological reagents) may provide the initial step for generation of data that may help in the execution of subsequent the definitive tests at a facility devoted to the in-depth analysis of biological samples.

Remember that the creation of a field test station does not obviate strict adherence to all safety rules. To the contrary, all personnel involved in preparing biological specimens suitable for rapid "at-the-office" microscopy must adhere strictly to all precautionary and safety measures in order to prevent contamination of staff and environment. Such precautions may demand wearing face shields, masks, gowns, and, at all times, gloves. Moreover, the space used for such procedures must be clearly marked as a biohazard environment and access to it should be restricted. **FINALLY, ALL WORK INVOLVING BACTERIAL CULTURES MUST BE PERFORMED AT SPECIALIZED FACILITIES (STATE OR FEDERAL).**

SPECIMEN COLLECTION: GENERAL RULES

Standard precautions (gloves, mask, gown) are mandatory during specimen collection in all cases of suspected exposure to biological warfare agents.

Blood

Standard Method

- Use sterile plastic syringes and needles that are completely dry.
- Draw a minimum of 4 to 5 cc
- If Vacutainer tubes are available, follow standard Vacutainer collection procedure
- If Vacutainer collection tubes are not available, use sterile, completely dry vials that can be securely sealed
- Remove the needle before transferring blood from the syringe to the vial
- Securely seal the space between the vial and the stopper with adhesive tape
- Label as indicated in the section below
- If the specimen cannot be delivered to the laboratory soon after collection, keep at 4°C (wet ice, frozen ice packs). Do not freeze

Filter Paper Method

This method simplifies transport. Body fluids other than blood can be collected using this method as well.

- If available, use standard collection cards; if not available, use strips of Whatman No. 1 paper
- Blood should be sampled from a finger (heels in infants) prick
- Clean the puncture site with 70% alcohol, then wipe completely dry with sterile gauze
- Puncture skin with a sterile lancet
- Wipe the first drop of blood away using sterile gauze
- To prevent hemolysis, do not squeeze the puncture site
- Touch the filter paper to the second droplet and soak it until the marked area on a standard card is filled; if card is not available, an area 0.6 to 1.6 cm in diameter must be filled
- Soak only one side of the paper
- Allow the sample to dry horizontally; do not allow contact between the specimen and other surfaces; avoid exposure to heat and sunlight.
- Do not refrigerate the sample
- Insert the dried sample into a clean plastic bag with a few grains of desiccant added, seal hermetically, and label as indicated in the section below
- Insert sample bag in a larger envelope provided with an appropriate label

Serum

- Acute sample
- At least 3 cc for suspected infectious pathogens; 20 cc for suspected toxins
- Freeze
- Label as indicated in the section below
- Insert in a larger envelope provided with an appropriate label

Sputum

- If possible, collect samples in the morning
- Optimally, 3 consecutive days of samples should be collected
- If sputum is scanty, 24-hour collection may be considered
- Use nebulized, hypertonic saline to induce sputum production in patients unable to bring it up
- Collect in wide-mouthed containers with lids that can be tightly sealed.
- Label as indicated in the section below
- Deliver to the laboratory as soon as possible
- If rapid delivery to the lab is impracticable, keep refrigerated at 4°C for maximum of 3 or 4 days

Tissue (Autopsy Material)

- Obtain multiple specimens, 25 to 50 g each
- Freeze for microbiology, toxicology, immunofluorescence polymerase chain reaction
- Formalin (4%) fix for histopathology; do not freeze
- Tissue specimens should include:
  - *Lung*
  - *Mediastinal lymph nodes*
  - *Spleen*
  - *Liver*
  - *Skin lesions if appropriate*

Nose and Throat Swabs

Nose

- Always take two swabs: one for a smear, one for bacterial culture
- Insert sterile cotton swab stick into the nasal opening to a depth of approximately 1 inch (2 to 3 cm)

- Scrub vigorously around the canal
- Perform the same procedure on the other side
- Place the swabs in a sterile, tightly sealed container
- Label as indicated in the section below

Throat

- Always take two swabs: one for a smear, one for bacterial culture
- With a sterile cotton swab stick, scrub the back of the throat, tonsils, and areas of inflammation or lesions
- Avoid touching the tongue or lips unless specifically required
- Place the swabs in a sterile tightly sealed container
- Label as indicated in the section below

Specimen Transport

Each specimen must be labeled with the patient's:
   – *Name*
   – *Age*
   – *Sex*
   – *Specimen type*
   – *Specimen number*
- Attach case investigation form for each specimen
- Collect ALL specimens related to a single case in one plastic bag and seal it securely
- Attach laboratory report in a separate plastic bag wrapped around the bag containing the samples
- Attach a form that establishes the chain of custody in strong and unequivocal terms
- Place the bag in a sturdy outer container (preferably plastic) and surround the bag with absorbent material that will absorb eventual leaks
- Seal the outer container securely with tape
- Place the container with samples into an insulated transport carrier and assure that the samples are kept cool by placing ice packs, wet ice, or dry ice (depending on the nature of the specimen) between the inner wall of the carrier and the sample container
- Affix the required biohazard labels to the outer surface of the carrier
- Ship by the most expeditious means available

PLAGUE SPECIMENS

All precautionary measures (gloves, mask, splash shield, gown) are mandatory for personnel dealing with plague specimens.

Bubo Aspiration

- Sterilize the site with tincture of iodine
- Use 10- or 20-cc syringe with 18/19 gauge needle
- Draw a few cc saline into the syringe
- Puncture the bubo and apply suction
- If aspiration produces no fluid, inject saline into the bubo, then draw again
- Transfer the contents of the syringe into a sterile tube (e.g., Vacutainer)
- Securely seal the seam between the tube and the stopper with tape
- Label the tube with patient's:
  - *Name*
  - *Age*
  - *Sex*
  - *Specimen type*
  - *Specimen number (if appropriate)*
  - *Date and time of collection*
- Transfer to appropriate laboratory

Sputum Collection

- Collect sputum in a sterile, wide-mouthed container
- Close the cap securely and seal with tape
- Label the container

SMALLPOX SPECIMENS

Vesicular or pustular fluid specimens from patients suspected of having smallpox must be collected by personnel vaccinated the same day or recently. All precautionary measures (gloves, mask, face shield, gown) are mandatory.

Collection

- Open the lesion with the blunt edge of a scalpel
- Collect the fluid on the cotton swab (Q-tip)
- Collect swabs with forceps
- Deposit the sample in a Vacutainer tube and tightly seal the junction between the tube and the stopper with adhesive tape
- Follow the general rules listed at the beginning of this chapter
- Contact appropriate local, state, and/or national public health authorities (relevant telephone numbers appear in Chapter 9) regarding shipment of samples

VACCINATION

Vaccination is typically performed using a sterile, bifurcated inoculation needle.

- Insert the needle into the ampule of reconstituted vaccine (upon removal, a droplet of liquid sufficient for vaccination will be held between the two prongs)
- Hold the needle perpendicular to the upper arm skin of the patient, with your wrist resting comfortably against the arm of the patient below the intended vaccination site (biceps muscle)
- Without moving your wrist from the patient's arm, perform 15 rapid, vigorous, perpendicular strokes within an area approximately 5 mm² of the patient's upper arm skin. The strokes are to be performed by pivoting your hand at the wrist. Blood should appear at the inoculation site within 15 to 30 seconds
- Wipe excess vaccine from the inoculation site with a gauze swab
- Discard the swab into a hazardous material receptacle. The receptacle should be clearly marked with a *biohazard* **sign**
- To prevent accidental touching and transferring of the virus to other parts of the body, cover the site with a loosely applied bandage
- Approximately 3 days following vaccination, a red papula will appear at the inoculation site. Two days later it will become vesicular. By the seventh day, a characteristic whitish, umbilicated, multiocular pustule containing turbid lymph will appear. Erythematous areola surrounding such Jennerian pustule may expand during the subsequent 3 days. The pustule will ultimately dry forming a dark crust that will detach itself in approximately 3 weeks
- Regional lymphadenopathy and fever are common side effects of vaccinia inoculation. In 70% of inoculated children, temperatures of 39°C (100°F) may be present for <24 hours between days 4 and 14 following vaccination

USEFUL MICROSCOPY TECHNIQUES

SMEAR PREPARATION

- Always wear gloves that fit! Gloves of the wrong size commonly cause accidental cuts
- Wear a mask
- Handle microscope slides by their edges, holding firmly
- Avoid handling slides by their corners — slides break easily
- Label slides with a soft lead pencil or an indelible ink pen
- Always perform all procedures over a bench
- Avoid moving slides with potentially highly contagious specimens away from the bench
- Avoid creating aerosols when air drying slides:
  - *Dry slides by placing them horizontally, away from air currents, dust, and possible contamination by insects*
  - *NEVER WAVE A SLIDE IN THE AIR IN AN ATTEMPT TO DRY IT!*

Blood Smear Preparation

- Perform finger stick (heel stick in infants)
- Squeeze the puncture site gently and place a single drop of blood approximately 1 to 2 cm from the end of a clean glass microscope slide
- Place the slide with the droplet firmly on a bench
- Inspect another clean (spreader) slide, make certain that its edges are perfectly smooth and free of nicks and indentations
- Place the short edge of the spreader slide against the surface of the blood slide at about a 45° angle, approximately 5 mm in front of the blood droplet (i.e., toward the longer end of the slide). The angle should appear between the spreader and the shorter end of the blood slide
- Move the spreader slide slowly without changing its angle until it makes contact with the droplet
- The droplet will rapidly spread along the contact line between the spreader and the blood slide
- When the contact line is fully covered with blood, immediately push the spreader in a single smooth movement toward the long end of the blood slide without changing the angle of the spreader

- The thickness of the resulting blood film depends on the speed of spreader movement. The faster the movement, the more even film and the better quality of the slide for microscopy
- The resultant film should be approximately 3 cm long, with the feathered end situated away from the original position of the droplet.
- Fix the smear in absolute methanol for 3 minutes if required because of transport or delay in microscopy
- Air dry the slide and label it with:
  - *Patient name*
  - *Date*
  - *Sequential slide number if relevant*
- Do not allow aerosols to form during the process of drying slides

Sputum Smear Preparation

- Place a clean microscope slide (sample slide) firmly on a bench
- Using a clean glass rod place a few droplets of the sputum on the sample slide and spread the droplets to produce an even film
- Air dry the slide
- Fix the slide in absolute methanol for 3 minutes
- If a thin smear is wanted, use the procedure cited earlier for a thin blood smear
- Do not allow aerosols to form during the process of drying slides

MICROSCOPY STAINS

No light microscopy stain provides the means of definitive identification of a pathogen. The clues may be very convincing, particularly when combined with the clinical picture, and thus useful in defining immediate forms of treatment. However, only cultures and more specific identification methods will provide definitive answers and definitive treatment approaches.

Gram Stain

Gram stain is the standard for the examination of specimens suspected to contain bacteria. The diagnosis based on examination of Gram-stained specimens is presumptive only, and requires confirmation by more specific methods (culture, polymerase chain reaction, etc.). Gram stain provides distinctive anatomical features, e.g., shape (cocci, bacilli) and arrangement (single organisms, clusters, chains), that provide strong clues to the nature of the infecting agent.

Results

- Gram-positive organisms: blue/black or purple
- Gram-negative organisms: pink/red
- Other structures (if pertinent):
  - *Nuclei: red*
  - *Collagen: shades of green*
  - *Red blood cells: shades of green*
  - *Cytoplasm: color varies*

Requirements

- Lillie's crystal violet (0.5%):
  - *Crystal violet: 2 g*
  - *Ammonium oxalate: 0.8 g*
  - *Ethanol (95): 20 ml*
  - *Distilled water: 80 ml*
- Gram's iodine (1%)
  - *Iodine: dissolve 1 g in small amount of water, then add remainder*
  - *Potassium iodide: 2 g*
  - *Distilled water: 300 ml*
- Safranine (0.5%)

Procedure

- Cover slide with Lillie's crystal violet solution for 1 minute
- Hold the slide downward, rinse briefly in tap water
- Pour Gram's iodine, allowing it to flow downward along the surface of the slide for 2 minutes
- Rinse briefly in tap water
- Differentiate in acetone **1 or 2 seconds** by holding the slide downward and pouring the acetone over the slide from the upper end
- Wash thoroughly in running tap water, then check the stain under a microscope. The background should NOT be purple
- Counterstain 30 seconds with safranine
- Rinse in water and dry
- Do not allow aerosols to form during the process of drying slides

Giemsa Stain (Wright or Wright–Giemsa Stain)

Giemsa stain can be used to detect plague bacteria ("safety-pin" bipolar staining) and, curiously, **smallpox**. In the latter case, aggregations of variola virus particles (Guarnieri bodies) show as reddish, hematoxylino-philic inclusions in the cytoplasms of cells from vesicular scrapings. Giemsa stain is available commercially (e.g., Fisher, Merck, etc.).

Results

- Plague: short, fat coccobacilli with bipolar "safety pin" staining patterns
- Smallpox: Guarnieri bodies (reddish cytoplasmic inclusions)
- Other structures
    - *Nuclei: blue/purple*
    - *Acidophils: pink/red*
    - *Basophils: blue*
    - *Eosinophils: orange/red*
    - *Mast cells: purple*
    - *Parasites: blue/dark blue*

Requirements

- Phosphate buffer (Sorensen):
    - *Stock A: 0.2 M sodium dihydrogen orthophosphate ($NaH_2PO_4H_2O$, MW 156); dissolve 3.12 g in 100 ml distilled water*
    - *Stock B: 0.2 M disodium hydrogen orthophosphate (Na_2HPO_4); dissolve 2.83 g in 100 ml distilled water*
    - *Mix 25.5 ml of A with 13.3 ml B; add distilled water to TOTAL 100 ml; the resulting pH will be 6.8*
- Giemsa stain stock:
    - *Mix 7.36 g Giemsa stain powder in 500 ml glycerol*
    - *Heat to 50°C (120°F) in a water bath for 30 minutes, stirring periodically*
    - *Allow to cool to room temperature*
    - *Add 500 ml methanol*
    - *Mix; filter through No. 1 Whatman paper*

Procedure

- Fix the smear slide in methanol for 5 minutes
- Dilute Giemsa stain stock with pH 6.8 buffer mix at 1:10 in a Coplin jar; if Coplin jar is unavailable, use a small beaker
- Place the slide in the Coplin jar containing the staining solution for 20 minutes

- If a beaker is used, make sure the smear surface is completely submerged in the staining solution
- Drain and dry at room temperature
- Do not allow aerosols to form during the process of drying slides

Gispen Silver Stain (Visualization of Cytoplasmic Smallpox Virus Aggregates)

Gispen's modified silver stain is in reality one of many existing modifications of Golgi's method based on the use of silver chromate as the staining medium. Although the use of the stain is quoted in most papers and books (including the present one) dealing with the detection of **variola** virus using laboratory methods, no references to the methodology are provided. For interested readers, the method is described in Geisert, E.E., Jr. and Updyke, B.V., Chemical stabilization of Golgi silver chromate impregnations, *Stain Technol.*, 52, 137, 1977. An equally good method is Grimelius stain (http://medlib.med.utah.edu/WebPath/HISTHTML/MANU-ALS/GRIMEL.PDF).

In practice and in the context of this manual, Gispen's stain and all other silver-based methods are unsuitable for field or rapid screening use. The specimens (vesicular scrapings) must be embedded in paraffin and then sectioned, mounted, and stained. The staining procedure, although relatively straightforward, requires some experience to yield reproducible results and eliminate artefactual silver grain precipitation.

Methylene Blue Stain (Plague Bacilli)

Methylene blue is probably the simplest stain to use to detect the presence of *Yersinia pestis*. However, since the stain is nonspecific, it provides only a very general indicator of the possible presence of plague bacilli.

Results

Bluish structures with the characteristic bipolar staining patterns suggest but do not definitvely confirm the presence of *Y. pestis*.

Requirements

The only reagent is aqueous methylene blue solution (1%) obtainable from a commercial supplier.

Procedure

- Use methanol fixed smears
- Immerse in the stain for 3 minutes using a Coplin jar or beaker
- Wash in tap water
- Dry
- Do not allow aerosols to form during the process of drying slides

Wayson Stain (Visualization of Plague Bacilli)

Wayson stain is a polychromatic differential stain suitable for the detection of *Yersinia* and *Pasteurella* species. **All *Y. pestis* organisms are Wayson-positive, but all Wayson-positive strains are not *Y. pestis.***

Results

Plague bacteria show as short, fat bacilli with bipolar staining producing the characteristic "safety pin" appearance.

Requirements

- A: basic fuchsin, 0.2 g (available commercially from Fisher, Merck, etc.)
- B: methylene blue, 0.75 g (available commercially from Fisher, Merck, etc.)
- Dissolve A and B in 20 ml 95% ethanol
- Filter the stain mix through No. 1 Whatman paper
- Add the stain to 200 ml 5% aqueous phenol solution
- Store in a dark place at room temperature

Procedure

- Use methanol fixed smears
- Immerse the slide in the stain for 5 to 10 seconds using either a Coplin jar or a beaker
- Wash in tap water
- Blot and dry
- Do not allow aerosols to form during the process of drying slides

6

PRECAUTIONARY MEASURES

DETECTION

General Factors Affecting Early Detection of Bioterrorism

Precautionary measures relevant to bioterrorism (or any other terrorist activity) involve operations based on a number of distinct but ultimately tightly interwoven plans. Clearly, the most important plan is prevention of the assault. It is also the most difficult aspect of activity because it has national and international ramifications. Development of appropriate intelligence resources, correlation of information gathered from a multiplicity of sources and agencies, creation of international intelligence collaboration and exchange, and ultimately the process of analysis of the available data are all essential aspects of the ability to predict the severity of a threat, its nature, and even the possible locations of the potential perpetrators of the terrorist act. Acquisition and analysis of intelligence data, while representing the most important proactive aspect of counterterrorism, remains the domain of agencies dedicated to intelligence gathering, military, and appropriate law enforcement organizations.

As long as the obtained information is tentative and nonverifiable, its immediate impact on healthcare operations and personnel is minimal. Nonetheless, even at that stage, a general warning may serve the important role of drawing the attention of both public health organizations and individual healthcare providers to the need to develop, revise, or test institutional and personal preparedness that will be required in the event the potential threat materializes.

Unlike the automated detection systems developed to identify chemical warfare agents, sensors for biological pathogens are largely experimental and available mainly to military personnel and, to a much lesser extent, to law enforcement agencies. Automated detection systems may be of limited value because of the nature of biological threats. Military use of biological weapons of mass destruction involves massive unleashing of pathogens by means of artillery and rocket barrages, motorboat or ground spraying devices, or aerial release. Acts of terror are more likely to be based on small-scale releases of relevant pathogens. Hence, the concentrations of agents released in a bioterrorist attack can be expected to be significantly lower than those one might encounter on a battlefield. Moreover, by the time the first patient presents, it is more than likely that environmental traces of the pathogen will be gone.

Portal of Entry Detection: Clinical and Epidemiological Factors

Despite our best intentions, not every letter, water fountain, and ventilation duct can be checked and protected. Because of such limitations, healthcare workers (paramedics, nurses, ER physicians) and family members represent the first level of our existing and potential bioterrorism detection systems and the first contacts with victims of biological warfare. As a result most of our active bioterrorism countermeasures are essentially retroactive. Hence, our ability to rapidly and definitively identify the involved pathogen and to implement preexisting response plans is critically dependent on the appropriate performance at the "entry portal" level.

In order to perform effectively as the most important early detection sensors of bioterrorism-related events, healthcare workers **must be familiar with the essential clinical signs of the relevant diseases.** Unfortunately, most **bioterrorism-relevant agents initially induce largely nonspecific signs, e.g., flu-like symptoms**. In some instances, however, a few easily ignored but very characteristic landmarks may be found by a vigilant physician, nurse, paramedic, or even an astute EMS dispatcher listening carefully to a telephone description. Close attention to such findings may help rapid institution of the effective treatment and may be vital in rapid and definitive identification of the threat. **VIGILANCE AT ALL LEVELS OF ENTRY INTO THE HEALTHCARE SYSTEM IS THE ESSENTIAL PREREQUISITE OF EARLY DETECTION.**

Clinical providers must be alert to several epidemiological factors that may be the indicators of a bioterrorism-related disease outbreak:

- Unusual presentation of what appears to be a common disease
- Unusual symptoms accompanying a common disease
- Large numbers of patients with similar unusual symptoms
- Failure to respond to standard therapy
- Disease caused by an uncommon agent
- Increased morbidity and mortality associated with a seemingly common disease

- Sudden increase in an endemic disease
- Clustering of patients with similar, often unusual symptoms around the same physical or temporal space (e.g., same building, proximity to air-conditioning vents and air ducts, etc.)
- Clustering of similar (unusual) disease events in geographically separated regions
- Increased numbers of dead animals that may precede or accompany appearance of unexplained symptoms in humans
- Presence of unusual, atypical, genetically modified, or "antiquated" experimental laboratory pathogen strains

PROTECTIVE CLOTHING

The U.S. Environmental Protection Agency standardized personal protective equipment at four different levels. Each level requires specific devices and garments:

Level A — Self-contained breathing apparatus (SCBA) and totally encapsulating chemical protective (TECP) suit. Level A provides the highest degree of protection including respiratory, mucous membrane, eye, and dermal protection.

Level B — Positive pressure respirator (SCBA or supplied air respirator [SAR]), nonencapsulated chemical-resistant garments, gloves, and boots. Level B provides the highest degree of respiratory protection with a degraded level of skin protection. Level B is relevant for operations in the hot zones of bioterrorism sites characterized by very high concentrations of the contagion.

Level C — Air-purifying respirator (APR), nonencapsulating chemical-resistant garments, gloves, and boots. Level C represents a degraded level of protection in comparison to Level B. It applies to operations in the hot zones of bioterrorism sites.

Level D — Level D encompasses standard universal precautions at the healthcare facility level. It affords no respiratory protection and minimal skin protection.

Activity Zones

The classical concept of operations concerned with the containment of hazardous material spills or releases into the environment (HAZMAT OPS) divides the territory affected by the spill is into three zones:

Hot zone — Area of primary contamination directly affected by the spill.

Warm zone — Area upwind from the spill. Contaminated victims, rescue personnel, and equipment may be brought to a warm zone for primary decontamination. If necessary, initial stabilizing treatment may be administered in this zone as well.

Cold zone — A completely uncontaminated area. Theoretically at least, a healthcare facility where the definitive treatment of victims is performed represents a cold zone.

A bioterrorist assault will most likely blur these classical distinctions, and the implementation of protective measures will depend to a large degree on the judgment and direct assessment of the contamination danger in relation to the specific circumstances.

A hot zone can be expected in the context of open warfare (battle front release or aerial attack on a civilian population) or as the consequence of a major accident at a biological weapons factory or a research facility. Probably the best example of the latter is the accidental release of anthrax at a Soviet site in Sverdlovsk in 1979.

In the most likely bioterrorism scenario, the hot zone will be highly transient. By the time the first victim is detected, the hot zone may have disappeared entirely since the released pathogens (with some exceptions such as anthrax spores in favorable environments, smallpox virus present in scabs, or T2 toxins) will be eliminated by contact with the environment (ultraviolet [UV] light, temperature, air, etc.). **However, buildings in which confirmed releases of a biological agent took place may be considered hot zones because of the possible continuous presence of the contagion. Similarly, a hospital room with a smallpox patient at the most infectious stage may be also considered a hot zone with respect to the rest of the facility.**

High flexibility in determining what constitutes warm zone is needed. Decontamination spaces, spaces where contaminated clothing and bedding are handled, and local laboratories growing bacterial and viral cultures may all be considered warm zones.

Even in declared cold zones, the risk of secondary infection may exist and an appropriate degree of alertness is necessary (see below).

Environments without Primary Contamination

Cold Zone

Personnel Involved in Patient Care

With a few possible exceptions (anthrax spores, smallpox virus in detached scabs, T2 toxins, etc.), the environmental contamination with the pathogen may typically be significantly reduced or absent by the time the first victims of a bioterrorist assault reach healthcare workers. Thus, unless pathogen release precedes presentation at the healthcare facility by a very short time, or direct contact with the contaminant is confirmed by victims or witnesses (e.g., in assassination attempts or via aerosol release in confined spaces), or traces of contamination (powder or liquid residues on clothing or skin) are present, the contact with the patient's clothing or skin will not pose significant danger of secondary contamination. **HOWEVER, PATIENTS PRESENTING WITH THE SIGNS OF PNEUMONIC PLAGUE, SMALLPOX, CRIMEAN–CONGO HEMORRHAGIC FEVER, AND EBOLA HEMORRHAGIC FEVER SHOULD BE CONSIDERED HAZARDOUS.**

As a safety measure, implementation of universal precautions and barrier nursing should be considered mandatory in all contacts with victims of a bioterrorist attack. It is also recommended that the universal precautions be implemented as a preemptive measure when definitive threats of such attacks are made.

Universal precautions require wearing of latex gloves (with a good, tight fit), surgical mask, face splash guard, and barrier gown. Surgical masks offer very little protection against most biological aerosols. It is unquestionably difficult to demand that healthcare workers wear air-purifying respirators equiped with highly efficient HEPA (high efficiency particulate air filters) in the environment of a vague and unspecified threat.

However, when an incident of a very recent large-scale aerosol exposure is reported or in situations where definitive detection of a highly contagious pathogen (e.g., smallpox, plague, or anthrax) is made, standard use of APRs (air purifying respirators) with HEPA filters is strongly advised in contacts with all patients presenting with suspicious or unusual symptoms.

As a standard rule, **it is better to be overcautious than infected. When unsure, assume the worst.**

Personnel Not Directly Involved in Patient Care

Personnel not directly involved in patient care face significant risk of infection, particularly the staff involved in **cleaning, removal of substances soiled by patient body fluids, feces, and secreta and diagnostic laboratory personnel.**

While not all biological agents are capable of causing secondary transmissions, anthrax bacilli will sporulate after a few hours' exposure to air and present potential risk for inhalational anthrax. Low temperature and lack of sunlight prolong the viability of plague bacilli, posing threats of secondary aerosolization and infection during postmortem examinations and disposal of remains. T2 toxins are very stable and, unless decontaminated, clothing of the affected patients poses a significant risk.

Therefore, depending on the nature of the agent, precautions ranging from universal through full respiratory and dermal protection measures must be considered as an aspect of the activities unrelated to direct patient care.

Warm Zone

Evidence from previous disasters indicates that many victims move directly from the hot zone to the nearest healthcare facility, typically the emergency room of the closest hospital. Hence, due to the stream of casualties bypassing field decontamination sites, the effective warm zone will shift to a hospital, clinic, or other designated treatment location. Such a situation will be typical in the event of a bioterrorism event involving a large area (e.g., dispersion of a pathogen from an aircraft). If such an event is strongly suspected or confirmed, **personnel in direct contact with the contaminated victims must wear respiratory protection.** Since the pathogens likely involved in such attack (with the exception of mycotoxins) will pose little or no danger of skin penetration, dermal protection by means of self-contained suits will not be necessary. Secondary aerosolization of residues left on the skin, hair, or clothes of victims will be insignificant under these circumstances.

IN SITUATIONS OTHER THAN LARGE-SCALE PATHOGEN EXPOSURE, STANDARD UNIVERSAL PRECAUTIONS AND BARRIER NURSING POSTURE WITH POWERED AIR-PURIFYING PROTECTION (PAPR) AND HEPA FILTERS ARE RECOMMENDED.

WHERE LARGE-SCALE EXPOSURE TO A BIOLOGICAL WARFARE AGENT IS STRONGLY SUSPECTED OR CONFIRMED, BE ALERT TO THE PRESENCE OF POWDERS, LIQUIDS, LIQUID DROPLETS, OR STAINS THAT MAY INDICATE CONTINUING PRESENCE OF THE CONTAMINANT. IF LIQUID CONTAMINATION IS NOTICED, AND AS A PRECAUTION AGAINST EXPOSURE TO T2 TOXINS (DISPERSED AS LIQUIDS OR MISTS), FULL DERMAL PROTECTION (NONENCAPSULATING SUITS) WITH HEPA FILTERS ATTACHED TO PAPRS IS RECOMMENDED.

Environments with Primary (Possibly Life-Threatening) Contamination

Hot Zone

A hot zone is an area directly affected by the release of the pathogen. Hot zones can exist outdoors (aircraft release of a pathogen) or indoors (release via ventilation ducts, mailed powders, explosions, or spray devices).

OPERATIONS IN A HOT ZONE REQUIRE FULL DERMAL AND RESPIRATORY PROTECTION. THE USE OF FULLY ENCAPSULATING PROTECTIVE GARMENTS AND SELF-CONTAINED OR SUPPLIED AIR RESPIRATORS IS MANDATORY. Both forms of protection are cumbersome, rapidly induce heat stress, and may limit the ability to communicate.

Apart from emergency medical services personnel in the field, it is unlikely that the majority of healthcare personnel will be exposed to activities in a hot zone. However, it is desirable that all emergency medical personnel including those in healthcare facilities become familiar with using uncomfortable and rapidly exhausting protective equipment and working while wearing it. They may constitute operational manpower reserves in critical situations during which they will have no time to learn how to use such equipment.

DECONTAMINATION

Two readily available solutions are commonly used for decontamination:

- 0.5% hypochlorite solution = 1 part Clorox + 9 parts water
- 5% hypochlorite solution = undiluted Clorox (5.25% solution)

During the process of decontamination, the environmental concentrations of biological pathogens (microbial organisms and their toxins) are reduced below their infective/toxic levels, leaving the environment safe for future activities. Decontamination can be performed using:

Mechanical methods — Filtration of air and water; water flush.
Chemical methods — Decontaminating liquids, sprays, or gases some of which may already be toxic.
Physical methods — Different forms of heat (flame, steam) or radiation (ultraviolet, microwave, ionizing).

Biological agent decontamination involves three processes:

Disinfection — The concentration of the pathogen is reduced below the effective pathogenic level; may be ineffective against spores.
Sterilization — Microbial organisms and their spores are killed.
Biotoxin decontamination — Complete deactivation or reduction of environmental toxin concentrations below harmful levels.

Five levels of decontamination must be considered in the context of bioterror:

Decontamination of patients
Decontamination of clothing and bedding
Decontamination of equipment
Decontamination of spaces (rooms)
Decontamination of outdoor environment

Decontamination of Patients

Intact Skin Surfaces

- Flushing with copious amounts of soap and water is sufficient in most cases

- Hypochlorite solution (0.5%) should be used only in cases of extensive contamination
  - *Contact time is 10 to 15 minutes*
  - *It may facilitate subsequent reinfections*

Eyes

- Remove contact lenses
- Rinse eyes with massive amounts of noncontaminated (sterile) water or saline for 15 minutes

Wounds

- Explore wounds with instruments, not with fingers
- Debride wounds using **no-touch techniques**
- **Do not use 0.5% hypochlorite solution to decontaminate:**
  - *Eyes (it causes corneal opacities)*
  - *Abdominal and thoracic wounds; complications are likely*
  - *Wounds that expose brain or spinal cord*
  - *Use saline, hydrogen peroxide, or other irrigation solutions instead of hypochlorite on such wounds*
- Use 0.5% hypochlorite solution on noncavity wounds:
  - *Apply to the wound for 5 minutes*
  - *Remove using suction*
  - *Collect into a disposable container; the fluid will be nonhazardous within 5 minutes*
  - *Irrigate the wound with saline*
- Insert removed tissue fragments, small pieces of clothing, etc., into a container decontaminated with 0.5% hypochlorite solution

Decontamination of Clothing and Bedding

- Immersion in 5% hypochlorite solution for 30 minutes
- Undiluted Clorox (5.25% hypochlorite solution) may be used
- Hypochlorite is an oxidant; it is destructive to fabrics
- If hypochlorite decontamination is impractical, consider incineration

HYPOCHLORITE THAT HAS BEEN ALLOWED TO DRY MUST NOT BE AUTOCLAVED OR DRY HEATED BECAUSE:

Organic material (cloth) + oxidizer (hypochlorite) + heat = explosion

Decontamination of Equipment

- Disposables:
  - *Soak overnight in **1% hypochlorite, 10% formalin, or 3% Lysol***
  - *Discard with garbage marked "Biohazard"/incinerate*
- Contaminated glassware:
  - *Place in a metal box or bucket*
  - *Place the container in the autoclave*
  - *Decontaminate by autoclaving*
- Surgical instruments:
  - *Method 1: immersion in 5% hypochlorite for 30 minutes:*
    - Rinse thoroughly in water
    - Oil surfaces and movable joints lightly; hypochlorite corrodes metals
    - Wipe with a cotton cloth
    - **Sterilize in dry heat at 160°C (~320°F) for 2 hours;** can be performed in an electric oven with a thermostat
  - *Method 2: immersion in 5% hypochlorite for 30 minutes:*
    - Rinse thoroughly in water
    - Autoclave at 125°C (~260°F) for ≥20 minutes (depending on volume) at 1 to 1.5 atm (15 to 22 lbs/inch^2) overpressure
    - If needed, lightly oil the surfaces and joints with sterile mineral oil
    - Wipe surfaces clean with sterile cloth.
  - *Method 3: red heat or flaming*
    - This is the method of last resort and should be considered only under extreme conditions. Only the operating surfaces (cutting edges, tips of blades, etc.) can be sterilized this way.
    - Use a gas burner
    - Hold the appropriate end of the instrument in the blue part of the flame cone for several seconds
    - Move the instrument slowly up and down
    - Pass the adjacent part of the instrument rapidly through the flame cone, allowing it to heat up
    - Place instrument on a sterile surface; allow to cool before use

Decontamination of Spaces (Rooms)

Space decontamination is typically performed by fumigation with antimicrobial vapors and gases or exposure to ultraviolet (UV) light. Ionizing radiation, while capable of killing microbial organisms and their spores, is impractical.

Decontamination of large spaces (office buildings, hospital buildings or floors, or private houses used to quarantine infected members of a household) is typically a complex endeavor and is best left to specialist decontamination teams. Limited scale space decontamination can be performed using either UV light or simple fumigation with formaldehyde.

Ultraviolet Light

Since UV light deactivates viruses, bacteria, and fungi, it is used in decontamination of air locks, patient rooms, and laboratory spaces.

- UV light can cause burns readily and proper precautions must be in place when this form of radiation is used. In spaces occupied for extended periods, UV lights should extinguish automatically when full spectrum lights are turned on
- UV light has little penetrating power. Hence, the surface of the UV lamp must be kept clean of dirt and dust that significantly reduce its efficiency
- **UV lamps lose their efficiency with time** and performance must be periodically checked using a UV meter or measuring strip

Formaldehyde (Formalin) Fumigation

This method is suitable for decontamination of relatively small rooms, laboratory spaces suspected of contamination, and similar spaces. When used with UV light, formaldehyde may provide an interim measure for decontamination of rooms vacated by infected patients. **FORMALIN IS A POWERFUL, HARMFUL RESPIRATORY IRRITANT AND A CARCINOGEN.**

- Seal all windows and doors with brown paper and adhesive tape.
- Pour 500 ml formalin and 1000 ml water into a pan
- Boil the mixture using a spirit lamp, gas burner, or electrical cooking plate
- Extinguish boiling device when very little fluid remains in the pan.
- Seal the exit door
- On the following day, open the door and place a piece of lint soaked in ammonia on the table to neutralize the excess of formalin present in the room

Decontamination of Outdoor Environment

The impact of natural outdoor elements (UV radiation, oxygen, temperature, etc.) will lead to a relatively rapid deactivation of biological pathogens. Hence, the need for outdoor environment decontamination will be highly unlikely in the context of a bioterrorist event. Terrain decontamination is costly and should be left to specialized decontamination units. If necessary, spraying with oily substances to prevent secondary aerosolization and the use of chlorine–calcium or lye may be considered.

TRIAGE

Triage of victims is frequently an inherent element of activities following a mass casualty incident. An act of bioterrorism may necessitate implementation of effective triage as well. Several standard approaches based on victim tagging have been developed. The most common approach is color tagging:

Green: healthy
Yellow: delayed treatment
Red: immediate treatment
Black: moribund/pain relief

Geometric figure or letter tagging (several forms) can easily lead to confusion. Tags must be attached prominently and securely with no possibility of being lost or misplaced accidentally.

Triage can induce significant stress and demands very difficult decisions that must be made rapidly and without hesitation. The use of simple classification and identification methods may help, at least partially, in alleviating the immediate emotional burden of making such decisions. However, in order to be efficient, triage methods must be:

■ Frequently practiced under realistic conditions
■ Uniformly practiced within the affected area
■ Clearly understood and followed by all involved personnel at the affected area
■ Clearly understood by personnel of all receiving facilities

PATIENT TRANSPORT

The majority of infections relevant to bioterrorism cannot be transmitted from person to person. However, standard precautions should be maintained while transporting patients suspected of being exposed to or diagnosed with anthrax, smallpox, plague, botulism, and tularemia. **It is also recommended, particularly during ambulance transport, that patients infected with smallpox, plague, and hemorrhagic fevers be provided with surgical face masks to reduce the danger of droplet dispersal.**

As a rule, the movement of patients with bioterrorism-related infections should be limited as much as possible and be dictated only by the necessities of patient decontamination and care. Movement within healthcare facilities should take place along predetermined routes that will eliminate the possibility of accidental contamination of cold zones and of unaffected patients.

HANDLING OF CONTAMINATED MATERIAL

Handling of contaminated material such as clothing and bed linen poses the danger of secondary aerosolization and infection. Standard precaution rules must be observed and the personnel should wear air-purifying respirators (APRs) with HEPA filters. Full dermal protection (nonencapsulating garments) may be considered, particularly in the presence of T2 toxins, weaponized anthrax spores, and materials contaminated with body fluids and excreta of patients with smallpox, plague, and certain hemorrhagic fevers.

Before transfer to the decontamination site or the incineration site, contaminated materials must be double bagged, with the bags securely tied. As an additional precaution, the outer surfaces of the bags may be sprayed with 0.5% hypochlorite solution. The transfer should take place along the previously established routes that will not cross clean areas or areas where decontaminated or uncontaminated patients and personnel may be present. Handling of laboratory specimens has been discussed in the preceding section.

HANDLING OF DECEASED VICTIMS

The problem of handling the bodies of victims of a bioterrorist attack represents a highly complicated arena involving ethical, legal, and religious issues. From the most simplistic point of view, the bodies of deceased victims found in a hot zone may present significant hazards, particularly if exposed to large concentrations of pathogens such as T2 toxins. Hence, the bodies may need to be treated as any other source of secondary contamination and as a threat to personnel and the rest of the population. The emotional impact of such an approach, particularly after the danger has been eliminated, may be very strong and incompatible with the rationalization implemented during the attack. While a thorough discussion of these highly complex problems is beyond the scope of the manual, this and other aspects of dealing with mass casualties after a chemical or biological terrorist attack demand very careful analysis and development of adequate plans in preparation for such events.

Most likely, however, even a well-orchestrated act of bioterrorism that would simultaneously involve multiple and widely separated sites would not produce extremely large numbers of simultaneous victims. The sophistication of pathogen-dispersing technology required, and the need for adequate saturation of the environment with an agent to assure the required infection potency despite continuing degradation by environmental factors (sunshine, temperature, presence of oxygen, etc.) mitigate against such scenarios. Contrary to an attack with chemical weapons, most events would be associated with a number of warm zones concentrated around treatment facilities rather than the classical hot zones. Deaths would be staggered because of dissimilar time courses of the disease among the affected persons. Even with a pathogen that can be transmitted from person to person, it is unlikely that the mortality would overwhelm the existing capacity for dignified burial or cremation of the deceased.

While healthcare and mortuary personnel involved in burials should implement universal precautions, the danger of secondary contamination will be limited. Importantly, once interred, the bodies will not present any further threat because environmental factors will contribute to very rapid elimination of the pathogen. Cremation of the bodies will result in efficient elimination of the potential for the secondary outbreaks of the disease.

7

PERSONNEL ISSUES RELEVANT TO BIOTERRORISM

PERSONNEL ISSUES

In similarity to all other disasters, acts of bioterrorism will amplify inadequacies stemming from poor preparedness. However, bioterrorism involves an assault with the most elusive and invisible weapons that inflict damage in a seemingly sudden and random manner. The fear induced by biological weapons is compounded by the fact that, based on widely accessible information provided by the media, a relatively innocuous sickness occurring during a period of declared attack threat will appear to a lay person as a very lethal disease caused by the pathogen introduced by bioterrorist. Hence, the news or even a rumor of a bioterrorist attack will cause a rapid and substantial increase in the number of visits to healthcare facilities by patients with essentially insignificant complaints, or those simply requiring psychological support and reassurance from medical personnel.

The explosive growth in the patient overload (that is already typical of the majority of emergency departments and walk-in clinics) created by an act of bioterrorism will put major strain on both personnel and materiel resources. Importantly, without appropriate prior planning and preparation, such strain is likely to result in a rapid decline of the efficiency of medical responses at both prehospital and hospital levels, followed by an unavoidable decline in the quality of the care provided.

It is necessary to realize that performance degradation among unprepared organizations consequent to a bioterrorist attack need not be related to the number of casualties. Even a small number of arriving or potential victims may significantly affect operations performed routinely due to the necessity for the continuously elevated state of medical alert, the need to introduce and maintain a number of precautionary measures, the requirement to create and maintain quarantine space, and even the need to modify logistical operations (e.g., patient, laundry, and food transport, etc.) that may require clear separation of "clean" and "contaminated" traffic.

Continued operations at the enhanced vigilance posture will ultimately result in considerable stress of the affected personnel. Imposition of strict quarantine conditions will magnify such stress considerably. Quarantine will freeze the number of immediately available medical personnel at the level existing immediately prior to the imposed movement restriction. As a result, a fixed number of increasingly tired and anxious but unrelieved staff will be forced to deal with a rapidly elevating number of affected victims.

Analysis of military operations conducted under very high levels of stress shows that prolonged exposure to fear, physical and mental exhaustion, and undiminished operational tempo lead frequently to the demoralization and collapse of untrained or unprepared units. Similar conditions are likely to apply to medical facilities operating under facility-wide quarantine conditions. Hence, a relatively rapid operational breakdown is a very strong possibility. If similar conditions occur at a number of other facilities within the same region, a major failure of medical countermeasures will take place endangering the entire disease containment effort. Clearly, while the logistic elements (stockpiling of pharmaceuticals and vaccines, equipment, support supplies, etc.) are essential, **the effective preplanning and preparation of the solutions to the personnel issues are pivotal for the success of managing the outcome of a bioterrorist assault.** All plans must be highly flexible and agent- and event-contingent rather than general. For example, smallpox will require different measures from tularemia; aerial release of anthrax spores will produce different problems from mail dissemination). **It is very difficult to introduce or execute, particularly by personnel without appropriate operational experience, any modifications to preexisting plans once a catastrophic event begins to evolve. Hence, the personnel readiness preparations must incorporate plans for:**

- Adequate training and testing of preparedness
- Schedules for double-shifting
- Temporary recruitment of additional medical, nursing, and paramedic staff from existing pools (e.g., retired personnel, personnel in training, volunteers from other regions)
- Recruitment of additional technical personnel
- Engagement of lay volunteers
- Adequate stress relief of personnel
- Adequate and functional means of communication between quarantined personnel and their families

PSYCHOLOGICAL ISSUES

Terrorism, both national and international, creates a number of specific psychological problems among the personnel involved in dealing with its consequences and among the general public. The unpredictability, suddenness, lethality, and the numbers of existing and potential casualties consequent to terrorist attacks will result in stress induced by the ever-present uncertainty and fear.

Population Impact

The possibility that biological agents may be employed magnifies stress induced by the threat of a terrorist assault. In the popular view, biological weapons are inherently associated with the element of ghastly stealth — a contagious and lethal agent, invisible and almost undetectable, spreads surreptitiously and leads to the disruption of even the most basic forms of human interaction. In reality, with the salutary exception of smallpox, the majority of biological agents of mass destruction will present relatively well-contained dangers for the civilian population of a country that is not involved in warfare with a neighbor whose geographical proximity permits long-range dispersion of biological agents using military means of delivery.

The recent history of military operations in which biological weapons have been used (e.g., aerial dispersal of a variety of pathogens by the Imperial Japanese Army in Manchuria, the alleged incidents of trichothecene mycotoxin use in Southeast Asia) and the natural outbreaks of Ebola and smallpox in Africa and VEE in South America confirm the essential inefficiency of biological weaponry.

Rationalizations notwithstanding, the psychological pressure imposed by bioterrorism upon a peaceful and stable society that is unused to major outbreaks of infectious disease can be very intense. The seemingly chaotic initial attempts at the identification of the pathogen, marshaling of adequate resources, and the possibility of largely unpopular measures that may be introduced (e.g., quarantine, travel restrictions, enhanced presence of law enforcement and military units) will deepen anxiety about personal safety, the mistrust of the authorities will fuel rumors, and eventually lead to the possibility of civil unrest and disobedience. The consequent need to maintain adequate population control will divert critical resources away from the task of eliminating the underlying threat by containing it to the smallest area possible and providing maximum assistance to people already affected by the disease. The only means of preventing rapid escalation of the public response to the level of general panic is by providing **adequate, timely, and truthful information on the nature of the disease, the containment measures that are being introduced, the available means of treatment, and the means by which the**

general public may assist the authorities in preventing further spread of the disease.

Equally important are the prophylactic measures providing the general public with adequate information on the nature of bioterrorism, the nature of the agents that may be potentially involved, and the most sensible prehospital responses to possible contamination, of which rapid and copious use of soap and water may be the most essential! **Such information should be presented in a manner devoid of all typical sensationalism and implementing all available dissemination media.** In similarity to all other potential disasters that may involve large numbers of casualties (e.g., hurricanes, floods, or fires), engaging the broadest levels of the general public in clearly conceived countermeasures may be the most effective means of limiting the impact of a bioterrorist assault.

Responder Impact

Independent of the scale of a bioterrorist attack, the psychological pressures imposed upon first responders and prehospital and hospital healthcare providers will be significant. Because they represent the first level of contact with the victims, personnel of these services face the greatest possibility of contamination and infection. The need for constant vigilance, realization of the probable dangers, and concerns about personal safety may ultimately lead to the deterioration of individual psychological barriers and result in absenteeism. The occurrence of the latter will be most likely more prevalent among the workers unused to personal danger and the execution of their duties under life-threatening circumstances. Consequently, there is a possibility that certain aspects of medical care delivery may be impaired, especially if the threat persists over a long period of time.

Another likely effect of prolonged, high-intensity operations consequent to a major bioterrorism event will manifest as a slow erosion of the originally high level of alertness and vigilance that may lead to accidental exposure of healthcare personnel to otherwise easily avoidable dangers. **Appropriate and frequent training combined with continuous maintenance of adequate knowledge and skills are the only preparatory measures that can be instituted as the prophylactic means of preparing for real-life operations**. Unfortunately, this form of training is both expensive and disruptive because it requires intense use of all resources that would be necessary under real circumstances. Such training would also involve periodic interruption of all typical duties by the relevant personnel and produce additional difficulties. **As conceivable interim measures, education and certification similar to the certification courses in ALS, ACLS, or ACTLS may be considered.**

Psychological Support Measures

In similarity to the armed forces personnel in action, disaster recovery workers frequently suppress their own feelings and emotions, and concentrate on professional performance instead. Continuous activity in a highly stressful environment of multiple casualties, personal danger, and possible social tension will (also in similarity to the military personnel in combat) result in syndromes similar to battle fatigue or even combat shock. **STRESS DEBRIEFING AND COUNSELING ARE MANDATORY ELEMENTS OF ALL ACTIVITIES BOTH DURING AND AFTER RECOVERY FOLLOWING A BIOTERRORIST ATTACK OR ANY OTHER LARGE-SCALE DISASTER EVENT.**

Although frequently neglected, plans for and subsequent efficient implementation of psychological support for the involved personnel (first responders, EMS personnel, hospital staffs) are essential to the success of all disaster recovery operations. Both at the time of bioterrorist attack and during its aftermath, **implementation of effective community counseling and psychological support measures must be considered.** Grief caused by sickness and possible deaths of family members, possible economic losses, persistent personal anxiety, and a host of other factors may lead to the development of numerous cases of posttraumatic stress disorder that will negatively affect subsequent recovery of the community.

SECURITY ISSUES

One of the essential and frequently neglected aspects of counterterrorism activities is the problem of assuring the safety and security of healthcare facilities and their personnel whose effective functioning is essential for the delivery of required medical care. Hence, establishment of appropriate **security perimeters** around receiving facilities is essential in order to prevent unregistered entry of contaminated victims into clean areas or prevent entry of distressed family members who may interrupt methodical delivery of care by physical intervention or by persistent requests for information. While both types of intrusions are eminently understandable, their occurrence may exert a very significant negative impact on the overall performance of the staff whose critical role is, after all, the delivery of the most efficient help to as many victims as possible. Efficient security perimeters can be established by:

- Locking and posting guards at all auxiliary facility entrances
- Posting guards at the main casualty receiving doors (typically the emergency room or the main entrance)

- Posting guards at the ambulance entry to the staging area in front of the receiving station at the treatment facility
- Posting traffic controlling barriers and/or uniformed law enforcement officers at all vehicular access sites (streets) and within 500 yards from the staging area in front of the facility (typically the ambulance staging area in front of the emergency room)
- Establishing moving guard patrols within the facility
- Maintaining effective and functional communication with the control room with separate radio frequencies dedicated to security traffic and open to both the facility guards and law enforcement officers guarding access to the perimeter

SECURITY PERSONNEL MAY HAVE DIRECT CONTACT WITH CONTAMINATED OR INFECTIOUS VICTIMS OF THE ATTACK. HENCE, THEY MUST BE TRAINED AND EQUIPPED WITH THE APPROPRIATE PROTECTIVE DEVICES (RESPIRATORY PROTECTION). FURTHERMORE, DUE TO THEIR EXTREMELY SENSITIVE POSITIONS IN RELATION TO HIGHLY DISTRESSED VICTIMS, THEIR RELATIVES, INTRUSIVE MEDIA PERSONNEL, ETC., THE SECURITY PERSONNEL MUST BE APPROPRIATELY TRAINED IN DEALING WITH POTENTIALLY HIGHLY EMOTIONAL SITUATIONS IN A SENSITIVE, EMPHATIC, BUT NONETHELESS DECISIVE MANNER.

TRAINING ISSUES

Both national and state plans have been or are in the process of development outlining the nature and scope of responses to the threat or bioterrorist attack. Ultimately, all these plans are based on the ability of the base units — local hospitals, EMS, law enforcement, etc. — to perform in a manner that will allow rapid detection, characterization, containment, and elimination of a bioterrorism-related disease outbreak. Assuming that all other elements of readiness are in place (appropriate materiel, facilities, supplies, and knowledge), operational training is the most critical ingredient that will assure efficiency and success during real-life emergencies.

"Train as you fight, and fight as you train" is the daily mantra of the armed forces whose almost religious practice assures the success in the field. The ever-present threat of a chemical or biological terrorism attack must impose the same rule upon the healthcare system and also upon the law enforcement, fire fighting, and other agencies that will provide their immediate support. Hence, training covering medical responses to bioterrorism **must be frequent, realistic, and involve all branches of the relevant services**. It must also incorporate elements of unpredictability and randomness that will eliminate routine approaches to a very unpredictable problem, and that will eliminate complacency resulting from "doing a drill." As many disasters at sea have shown, complacency in the execution of lifeboat or firefighting drills always resulted in casualties that could have been easily avoided.

There is no doubt that realistic training can be highly disruptive to the routine activities of a hospital or an EMS unit. It can also be quite expensive. For both reasons, it is unpopular. Yet, bioterrorism presents challenges that exceed those facing healthcare personnel under normal circumstances.

The most important of those challenges is the always present element of **very significant personal risk**. While contamination with a deadly agent is always possible during any medical encounter, the virulence and lethality of the diseases most likely to be encountered in the context of bioterrorism multiply this risk many times. The risk can be minimized by **intensive training in the rigorous implementation of personal safety and through habituation of healthcare personnel to performing their activities while wearing protective devices that may be physically uncomfortable, reduce manual dexterity, or impair vision.** Familiarity with personal precautionary measures and procedures, and the understanding of their **practical as opposed to theoretical role obtained through reasonably frequent practical training** will be the most critical contributor to reducing reluctance and fear among healthcare personnel facing the reality of a chemical or biological assault.

The second challenge is **the environmental threat** to the healthcare facility. Again, **vigorous training of medical teams** can be the only answer to preventing nosocomial contamination and possible closure of the entire facility. **Frequent and realistic practice** by employees of the **admission procedures, isolation, waste transport and disposal, handling of clothing and bed linen, etc.**, is required. In addition, logistical approaches to such issues as a rapid increase in the demand for specific drugs, supplies, or devices must not only be planned, but **trained, preferably in the context of events that occur suddenly and unpredictably, i.e., in a manner similar to a terrorist attack.** It is a widely known fact that plans developed and theoretically ready for implementation in a mass casualty event have failed **due to the inconsistent or even faulty training in practical implementation prior to the real-life event.**

A host of other issues are common not only for the bioterrorist attacks but for practically all events that may result in mass casualties, e.g., natural disasters, large-scale highway, rail, air, or sea traffic accidents, or environmental releases of massively toxic substances. Preparation for such events requires the development of effective communications with other healthcare facilities and organizations at both regional and national levels, functional operational liaison and operational communications between healthcare facilities and EMS, law enforcement, firefighter units, and a properly functioning public relations apparatus capable of providing clear and truthful information to the affected population. All these elements will play critical roles in a practical approach to a bioterrorist attack. **However, the readiness to implement such procedures can be attained and maintained only in a direct relation to the adequacy, frequency, and realism of the relevant training**.

8

RESOURCES

All URL addresses were checked at the time the manuscript went to print. However, they change and do so without warning. Because the names of the institutions remain constant, the interested reader is encouraged to find the new address by using the name of the institution and any of the available Web search engines to find the new site.

FEDERAL, STATE, AND INTERNATIONAL ORGANIZATIONS

Air War College
http://www.au.af.mil/au/awc/awcgate/awc-hmld.htm

Armed Forces Institute of Pathology
http://www.afip.org/

Canadian Centre for Emergency Preparedness
http://www.ccep.ca/

CDC, Bioterrorism Preparedness and Response Branch
http://www.bt.cdc.gov/

CDC, Emergency Preparedness and Response Branch, Emergency Resources Site
http://www.cdc.gov/nceh/emergency/default.htm

CDC, Epidemic Intelligence Service
http://www.cdc.gov/eis/

CDC, National Center for Infectious Diseases
http://www.cdc.gov/ncidod/diseases/index.htm

CDC, Office of Health and Safety
http://www.cdc.gov/od/ohs/

Department of Defense, Office of the Deputy Assistant Secretary of
Defense for Counterproliferation and Chemical and Biological
Defense Programs DASD (CP/CBD)
http://www.acq.osd.mil/cp/

Department of Energy
http://www.dp.doe.gov/emergencyresponse/

Department of Health and Human Services (DHHS)
http://dhhs.gov/

DHHS, Office of Emergency Preparedness (OEP)
http://ndms.dhhs.gov/index.html

DHHS, Office of Emergency Preparedness, National Disaster Medical
System, Response Team Web Sites
http://ndms.dhhs.gov/Links/Team_Web_Sites/team_web_sites.html

DHHS, Office of Emergency Preparedness, Metropolitan Medical
Response System
http://www.oep-ndms.dhhs.gov/CT_Program/MMRS/mmrs.html

Department of Justice, Office for Domestic Preparedness
http://www.ojp.usdoj.gov/odp/

Department of Transportation, Office of Hazardous Materials Safety
http://hazmat.dot.gov/

EPA, Emergency Response Team
http://www.ert.org/

Federal Emergency Management Agency (FEMA)
http://www.fema.gov/

Department of Defense (DoD), Global Emerging Infections System
http://www.geis.ha.osd.mil/

DoD, Joint Service Chemical Biological Information System, Tracking System for Equipment Development
http://www.moxietraining.com/oshalinks/bioterrorism.htm

Lawrence Livermore National Laboratory
http://www.llnl.gov/nai/rdiv/rdiv.html

National Institutes of Health (NIH)
http://www.nih.gov/

National Institute for Occupational Safety and Health
http://www.cdc.gov/niosh/homepage.html

National Library of Medicine, Biodefense and Bioterrorism Information Resources
http://www.nlm.nih.gov/medlineplus/biodefenseandbioterrorism.html

U.S. Coast Guard, National Response Center
http://www.nrc.uscg.mil/index.htm

Occupational Safety and Health Administration
http://www.osha.gov/

DoD, Office of Counterproliferation and Chemical and Biological Defense
http://www.acq.osd.mil/cp/organization.html

Pan American Health Organization, Disaster and Humanitarian Assistance Office
http://165.158.1.110/english/ped/pedhome.htm

DoD, Program Director for Biological Defense Systems
http://www.sbccom.apgea.army.mil/RDA/pdbio/index.htm

State Health Department Web Sites
http://www.cdc.gov/search2.htm
http://www.phppo.cdc.gov/phtn/sites.asp

U.S. Army, Medical Command
http://www.armymedicine.army.mil/default2.htm

U.S. Army, Medical Research and Material Command
http://mrmc-www.army.mil/

U.S. Army, Medical Research Institute of Infectious Diseases
http://www.usamriid.army.mil/

U.S. Army, Office of the Surgeon General, Medical NBC (nuclear,
biological, chemical) Online Information Server
http://www.nbc-med.org/ie40/

U.S. Army, Soldier and Biological Chemical Command (SBCCOM)
http://www.sbccom.apgea.army.mil/

World Health Organization (WHO)
http://www.who.int/

FEDERAL AND STATE AGENCY REPORTS

GAO Report, Combating Terrorism, November 2000
http://www.gao.gov/new.items/d0114.pdf

Public Health Response to Biological and Chemical Terrorism, Interim
Planning Guidance for State Public Health Officials, CDC, July 2001
http://www.bt.cdc.gov/Documents/Planning/PlanningGuidance.PDF

Federal WMD Contingency Plan, United States Government Interagency
Domestic Terrorism Concept of Operations Plan
http://www.fbi.gov/publications/conplan/conplan.pdf

Biological and Chemical Terrorism: Strategic Plan for Preparedness and
Response, Recommendations of the CDC Strategic Planning Work-
group, April 21, 2000
http://www.cdc.gov/mmwr/preview/mmwrhtml/rr4904a1.htm

Recognition of Illness Associated with the Intentional Release of a
Biologic Agent, CDC, *MMWR*, October 19, 2001/50(41); 893-7
http://www.cdc.gov/mmwr/preview/mmwrhtml/mm5041a2.htm

Guidelines for Infection Control in Health Care Personnel, CDC, 1998
http://www.cdc.gov/ncidod/hip/guide/InfectControl98.pdf

Guidelines for Environmental Infection Control in Healthcare Facilities,
2003
http://www.cdc.gov/ncidod/hip/enviro/guide.htm

Patient Handling Precautions for BT agents (WRAMC)
http://www.tdh.state.tx.us/bioterrorism/btmanag.pdf

Guidelines for Isolation Precautions in Hospitals, CDC
http://www.cdc.gov/ncidod/hip/isolat/isolat.htm

Guide for the Selection of Chemical and Biological Decontamination
  Equipment for Emergency First Responders, NIJ Guide 103-00
http://www.ojp.usdoj.gov/nij/pubs-sum/189724.htm

Interim Recommendations for Firefighters and Other First Responders
  for the Selection and Use of Protective Clothing and Respirators
  against Biological Agents, CDC, October 2001
http://www.bt.cdc.gov/DocumentsApp/Anthrax/Protective/
  10242001Protect.asp

Human Behavior and WMD Crisis/Risk Communication Workshop
  Report, December 11–12, 2000
http://www.dtra.mil/about/organization/finalreport.pdf

Public Information, A Primer on Health Risk Communication Principles
  and Practices, ATSDR
http://www.atsdr.cdc.gov/HEC/primer.html

Installation Preparedness for Weapons of Mass Destruction: Installation
  Commanders Blueprint, Department of the Army, May 2001
http://www.hqda.army.mil/acsimweb/fd/policy/
  fire/docs/handbook0420final.pdf

OSHA, Mail Handling Instructions
http://www.osha.gov/bioterrorism/anthrax/question5.html

OSHA, How To Prepare For Workplace Emergencies
http://www.govstar.com/tahoe/emr.nsf/0/A395B37358E5651C86256AD
  400463C0D?OpenDocument&Cat = Emergency v/Publications/
  Osha3088.pdf
or
http://www.osha-slc.gov/Publications/Osha3088.pdf

OSHA, Workplace Guidance for Anthrax Issues
http://www.osha.gov/bioterrorism/anthrax/matrix/index.html

Maryland Department of Health Bioterrorism Article Compendium
http://www.dhmh.state.md.us/eis6501/biotbiot.htm

BOOKS AND MANUALS

Biological Terrorism Response Manual, Rega, P., 2000
http://www.bioterry.com/About_the_Book.asp

Defense against Toxin Weapons, DoD
http://www.usamriid.army.mil/education/toxdefbook.pdf

Electronic Textbook of Dermatology
http://telemedicine.org/stamford.htm

e-Medicine World Medical Library
http://www.emedicine.com/emerg/cover.htm

FEMA, *State and Local Guide (SLG) 101: Guide for All-Hazard Emergency Operations Planning*
http://www.fema.gov

Defense Threat Reduction Agency
http://www.nbc-med.org/SiteContent/MedRef/OnlineRef/FieldManuals/datw/index.htm

Medical Department of the Army, Medical Aspects of Chemical and Biological Warfare
http://www.nbc-med.org/SiteContent/HomePage/WhatsNew/MedAspects/CWBWFMelectrv699.pdf

U.S. Army, MRIID, *Medical Management of Biological Casualties,* 3rd ed,, 1998
http://www.nbc-med.org/SiteContent/MedRef/OnlineRef/FieldManuals/medman/Handbook.htm

U.S. Army, Field Manual 8-284, *Treatment of Biological Warfare Casualties*, July 17, 2000
http://www.adtdl.army.mil/cgi-bin/atdl.dll/fm/8-284/fm8-284.pdf

DoD, Weapons of Mass Destruction (WMD) Handbook, JCS, J-3
http://www.homelanddefense.org/J3WMDHandbook.pdf

Virtual Naval Hospital
http://www.vnh.org/FM8284/

RELEVANT ORGANIZATIONS

American Academy on Veterinary Disaster Medicine
http://www.cvmbs.colostate.edu/clinsci/wing/aavdm/aavdm.htm

American Civil Defense Association
http://www.tacda.org/

American College of Emergency Physicians
http://www.acep.org/1,4634,0.html

American Academy of Family Physicians
http://www.btresponse.org/

American Academy of Pediatrics
http://www.aap.org/advocacy/releases/cad.htm

American College of Physicians/American Society of Internal Medicine
    (Palm-based data)
http://www.acponline.org/pda/index.html

American Society of Microbiology Bioterrorism Web Links
http://www.asmusa.org/pcsrc/bioprep.htm

Association for Professionals in Infection Control and Epidemiology
http://www.apic.org/educ

Federation of American Scientists, Chemical and Biological Arms
    Control Program
http://www.fas.org/bwc/

Federation of American Scientists, Agricultural Biowarfare and
    Bioterrorism Site
http://www.fas.org/bwc/agr/main.htm

International Society for Infectious Diseases Program for Monitoring
    Emerging Diseases
http://www.promedmail.org

RESEARCH ORGANIZATIONS

Center for Nonproliferation Studies, Monterey Institute for International
  Studies
http://cns.miis.edu/

Center for the Study of Bioterrorism and Emerging Infections, Saint
  Louis University School of Public Health
http://www.bioterrorism.slu.edu/

Chemical and Biological Defense Information Analysis Center (CBIAC)
http://www.cbiac.apgea.army.mil/

Chemical and Biological Arms Control Institute
http://www.cbaci.org/

DRUGS

Antibiotic Treatment Site Guide (Specifies for BT agents), Johns
  Hopkins Division of Infectious Diseases
http://www.hopkins-abxguide.org/

Drug and Vaccine Information Site (FDA)
http://www.fda.gov/cder/drugprepare/default.htm

Smallpox, Vaccine Recommendations of the Advisory Committee on
  Immunization Practices (ACIP), 2001
http://www.cdc.gov/mmwr/preview/mmwrhtml/rr5010a1.htm

BIOLOGICAL AGENTS

Anthrax, MMWR Guidelines Update, Miscellaneous Documents,
  November 2, 2001, Vol. 50, No. 43
http://www.cdc.gov/mmwr/preview/mmwrhtml/mm5043a1.htm

Anthrax, Clinical Photographs, Gorgas Course in Clinical Tropical
  Medicine
http://info.dom.uab.edu/gorgas/anthrax.html

Hemorrhagic Fevers: Consensus Recommendations, *JAMA*, 2002, 287,
  2391–2405
http://jama.ama-assn.org/cgi/content/full/287/18/2391

Plague: Consensus Recommendations, *JAMA* 2001, 283, 2281–2290
http://jama.ama-assn.org/cgi/content/full/283/17/2281

Smallpox: Consensus Recommendations, *JAMA*, 1999, 281, 2127–2137
http://jama.ama-assn.org/cgi/content/full/281/22/2127

Tularemia: Consensus Recommendations, *JAMA* 2001, 285, 2763–2773
http://jama.ama-assn.org/cgi/content/full/285/21/2763

Biological Agent Fact Sheets, APIC
http://www.apic.org/bioterror/agentsheets.cfm

CDC, Biological Agent Information
http://www.bt.cdc.gov/Agent/Agentlist.asp

Bioterrorism Disease Wall Chart
http://www.unc.edu/depts/spice/bioterrorism.html

CBW, Information
http://www.cbwinfo.com/

CDC, Electronic Publications and Documents
http://www.cdc.gov/ncidod/publicat.htm

*Diagnosis and Management of Foodborne Illnesses: A Primer for
    Physicians*, MMWR/CDC and AMA, January 26, 2001
http://www.cdc.gov/mmwr/PDF/rr/rr5002.pdf

National Library of Medicine Anthrax and Biological Warfare
    Information Resources
http://www.nlm.nih.gov/biodefenseandbioterrorism.html

Virtual Naval Hospital
http://www.vnh.org/FM8284/

PERIODICALS AND OTHER PUBLICATIONS

DHHS, *Agency for Toxic Substances and Disease Newsletter*
http://www.atsdr.cdc.gov/HEC/hsphhome.html

Air University Index to Military Periodicals
http://www.dtic.mil/search97doc/aulimp/main.htm

ANSER, *Homeland Security Bulletin*
http://www.homelandsecurity.org/

Applied Science and Analysis, Inc.
http://www.asanltr.com/

Archives of Dermatology: Cutaneous Manifestations of Biological
  Warfare
http://archderm.ama-assn.org/cgi/content/short/135/3/311

Arista Tek, HAZMAT Software
http://www.aristatek.com/

Biodefense Quarterly, Center for Civilian Biodefense Studies, Johns
  Hopkins University
http://www.hopkins-biodefense.org/pages/news/quarter.html

British Medical Journal
http://bmj.com/

U.S. Army, Soldiers and Biological Chemical Command, *CB Quarterly*
http://www.sbccom.apgea.army.mil/RDA/quarterly/index.htm

Chemical and Biological Information Analysis Center Newsletter
http://www.cbiac.apgea.army.mil/awareness/newsletter/intro.html

U.S. Army Center for Health Promotion and Preventive Medicine,
  CHPPM News Bulletin
http://chppm-www.apgea.army.mil/imo/ddb/dmd/DMD/NEWS.HTML

U.S. Army Chemical School, CML, *Army Chemical Review*
http://www.wood.army.mil/CHBULlETIN/Default.htm

Chemical and Biological Arms Control Institute, *Dispatch*
http://www.cbaci.org/dispatch.htm

CDC, National Center for Infectious Diseases, Emerging Infectious
  Diseases
http://www.cdc.gov/ncidod/eid/index.htm

Emergency Information Infrastructure Partnership Newsletter
http://www.emforum.org/eiip/news.htm

FEMA News Listing
http://www.fema.gov

Red Hat Publishing, Fire and Emergency Response Materials
http://www.redhatpub.com/

Department of the Army, *Hazardous Technical Information Service
Newsletter*
http://www.dscr.dla.mil/htis/

JAMA (especially archival bioterrorism section)
http://jama.ama-assn.org/

Journal of Homeland Defense
http://www.homelanddefense.org/

Journal of Homeland Security
http://www.homelandsecurity.org/journal/index.cfm

Journal of Terrorism and Political Violence
http://www.frankcass.com/jnls/tpv.htm

Military Medical Technology Online
http://www.mmt-kmi.com/

CDC, *Morbidity and Mortality Weekly Report* (*MMWR*)
http://www.cdc.gov/mmwr

National Fire and Rescue Magazine
http://www.nfrmag.com/

Nonproliferation Review, Center for Nonproliferation Studies, Monterey
Institute of International Studies
http://cns.miis.edu/pubs/npr/index.htm

Department of Justice, *Office for State and Local Domestic Preparedness
Support Bulletins*
http://www.ojp.usdoj.gov/odp/docs/bulletins.htm

OSHA, *Job Safety and Health Quarterly Magazine*
http://www.osha-slc.gov/html/jshq-index.html

Tempest Publishing (resources center section)
http://www.chem-bio.com

Centers for Disease Control Mailing Lists (multiple publications)
http://www.cdc.gov/subscribe.html

Chemical and Biological Arms Control Institute Dispatch Bulletin
(e-mail to request service)
http://www.cbaci.org/

U.S. Environmental Protection Agency (multiple list servers)
http://www.epa.gov/epahome/listserv.htm

Monterey Institute, Center for Nonproliferation Studies, *WMD Bulletin*
http://cns.miis.edu/research/cbw/index.htm

Natural Hazards Center, University of Colorado (consolidated list of
sources)
http://www.colorado.edu/hazards/sites/lists.html

Terrorism Research Center, *Information Bulletin*
http://www.terrorism.org/mailman/listinfo/realnews

Federal Medical Bulletin Service, *This Week in U.S. Medicine*
http://www.usmedicine.com/

Workers Education and Training Program, National Institute of
Environmental Health Sciences, National Institutes of Health
http://www.niehs.nih.gov/wetp/home.htm

DISCUSSION GROUPS

Chemical Doctrine List Server, U.S. Army Chemical School (go to
Chemical Doctrine and sign up per instructions)
http://confs.itcenter.org/

Daily Brief (Miscellaneous Emergency Management) Discussion List
http://groups.yahoo.com/group/DailyBrief

Dangerous Goods List Server: Storage and Handling Commercial
Products
http://www.onelist.com/subscribe/DangerousGoods

Department of Justice, Office of Domestic Preparedness List Server
email listproc@lists.aspensys.com.
(in the body of the message type subscribe _ your name)

Emergency Management Discussion List
http://groups.yahoo.com/group/emergency-management
To reach the Moderator:
emergency-management-owner@yahoogroups.com

Emergency Management Legislation List Server
Subscribe at: emlegislation-subscribe@yahoogroups.com
To reach the Moderator:
emlegislation-owner@yahoogroups.com

HAZMAT–WMD Discussion List
http://groups.yahoo.com/group/Hazmat-WMD

International Association of Emergency Managers Emergency
    Management Discussion List
http://www.iaem.com/

EQUIPMENT

Disaster Central (resource guide)
http://www.disaster-central.com/

CCS International (equipment)
http://www.spyzone.com/

Disaster-resource (online guide)
http://www.disaster-resource.com/

Domestic Preparedness (commercial site; conference and event listings)
http://www.domesticpreparedness.com/

First Responders.com (private web site for first responders)
http://wmdfirstresponders.com/

Isolation Systems Incorporated (air purifying systems)
http://www.hivroom.com/

Jane's Chem-Bio Web (requires paid subscription)
http://chembio.janes.com/

MITRETEK (WMD systems applications)
http://www.mitretek.org/mission/envene/nbc.html

TRAINING

DHHS and American College of Emergency Physicians, *Developing Objectives, Content, and Competencies for the Training of Emergency Medical Technicians, Emergency Physicians, and Emergency Nurses to Care for Casualties Resulting From Nuclear, Biological, or Chemical (NBC) Incidents,* Final Report
http://www.acep.org/library/index.cfm/id/2676.pdf

MedSMART, Inc. (mass simulation-based distributed medical training for first responders)
http://www.med-smart.org

St. Michael's Group (school and workplace security)
http://www.stmichaelsgrp.com/

EMERGENCY MANAGEMENT

Decon liability for first responders (EPA)
http://www.epa.gov/ceppo/pubs/onepage.pdf

MedicCom.Org, Toledo, Ohio Disaster Medical Assistance Team
http://mediccom.org/public/default.htm

National Center on Emergency Planning for People with Disabilities (no web site)
Email: NCEPPD@inclusioninc.com
Telephone: 202-546-4464, Ext. 201

National Voluntary Organizations Active in Disasters (NVOAD)
http://www.nvoad.org/

Emergency Information Infrastructure Partnership
http://www.emforum.org/

Emergency Net, Emergency Response and Research Institute
http://www.emergency.com/

NBC Industry Group
http://www.nbcindustrygroup.com/

9

FEDERAL AND STATE AGENCIES RELEVANT TO COUNTER-BIOTERRORISM

U.S. DEPARTMENT OF JUSTICE

Domestic Preparedness National Response Hotline (agencies only)
1-800-424-8802

FEDERAL BUREAU OF INVESTIGATION (FBI)
FIELD OFFICES

Albany, NY 12209
200 McCarty Avenue
518-465-7551

Albuquerque, NM 87102
415 Silver Avenue SW, Suite 300
505-224-2000

Anchorage, AK 99501
101 East 6th Avenue
907-258-5322

Atlanta, GA 30345
2635 Century Parkway NE, Suite 400
404-679-9000

Baltimore, MD 21244
7142 Ambassador Road
410-265-8080

Birmingham, AL 35203
2121 8th Avenue North, Room 1400
205-326-6166

Boston, MA 02108
One Center Plaza, Suite 600
617-742-5533

Buffalo, NY 14202
One FBI Plaza
716-856-7800

Charlotte, NC 28285
400 South Tryon Street, Suite 900
704-377-9200

Chicago, IL 60604
219 South Dearborn Street, Room 905
312-431-1333

Cincinnati, OH 45202
550 Main Street, Room 9000
513-421-4310

Cleveland, OH 44199
1240 East 9th Street, Room 3005
216-522-1400

Columbia, SC 29210
151 Westpark Boulevard
803-551-1200

Dallas, TX 75202
1801 North Lamar, Suite 300
214-720-2200

Denver, CO 80294
1961 Stout Street, Room 1823
303-629-7171

Detroit, MI 48226
477 Michigan Avenue, 26th Floor
313-965-2323

El Paso, TX 79912
660 South Mesa Hills Drive, Suite 3000
915-832-5000

Honolulu, HI 98850
300 Ala Moana Boulevard, Room 4-230
808-521-1411

Houston, TX 77008
2500 East T.C. Jester
713-693-5000

Indianapolis, IN 46204
575 North Pennsylvania Street, Room 679
317-639-3301

Jackson, MS 39269
100 West Capitol Street, Suite 1553
601-948-5000

Jacksonville, FL 32211
7820 Arlington Expressway, Suite 200
904-721-1211

Kansas City, MO 64105
1300 Summit Street
816-221-6100

Knoxville, TN 37902
710 Locust Street, Suite 600
423-544-0751

Las Vegas, NV 89104
700 East Charleston Boulevard
702-385-1281

Little Rock, AR 72211
10825 Financial Centre Parkway, Suite 200
501-221-9100

Los Angeles, CA 90024
11000 Wilshire Boulevard, Suite 1700
310-477-6565

Louisville, KY 40202
600 Martin Luther King Jr. Place, Room 500
502-583-3941

Memphis, TN 38120
225 North Humphreys Boulevard, Suite 3000
901-747-4300

Miami, FL 33169
16320 NW 2nd Avenue
305-944-9101

Milwaukee, WI 53202
330 East Kilbourn Avenue, Suite 600
414-276-4684

Minneapolis, MN 55401
111 Washington Avenue South, Suite 1100
612-376-3200

Mobile, AL 36602
One St. Louis Street, 3rd Floor
334-438-3674

New Haven, CT 06510
150 Court Street, Room 535
203-777-6311

New Orleans, LA 70113
1250 Poydras Street, Suite 2200
504-522-4671

New York, NY 10278
26 Federal Plaza, 23rd Floor
212-384-1000

Newark, NJ 07102
One Gateway Center, 22nd Floor
973-622-5613

Norfolk, VA 23502
150 Corporate Boulevard
757-455-0100

Oklahoma City, OK 73118
50 Penn Place, Suite 1600
405-290-7770

Omaha, NE 68114
10755 Burt Street
402-493-8688

Philadelphia, PA 19106
600 Arch Street, 8th Floor
215-418-4000

Phoenix, AZ 85012
201 E. Indianola Avenue, Suite 400
602-279-5511

Pittsburgh, PA 15219
700 Grant Street, Suite 300
412-471-2000

Portland, OR 97201
1500 Southwest 1st Avenue, Suite 400
503-224-4181

Richmond, VA 23228
111 Greencourt Road
804-261-1044

Sacramento, CA 95841
4500 Orange Grove Avenue
916-481-9110

Salt Lake City, UT 84111
257 East 200 South, Suite 1200
801-579-1400

San Antonio, TX 78205
615 East Houston Street, Suite 200
210-225-6741

San Diego, CA 92123
9797 Aero Drive
619-565-1255

San Francisco, CA 94102
450 Golden Gate Avenue, 13th Floor
415-53-400 [INCOMPLETE]

San Juan, PR 00918
150 Carlos Chardon, Room 526
787-754-000 [INCOMPLETE]

Seattle, WA 98174
915 Second Avenue, Room 710
206-622-460 [INCOMPLETE]

Springfield, IL 62704
400 W. Monroe Street, Suite 400
217-522-675 [INCOMPLETE]

St. Louis, MO 63103
2222 Market Street
314-231-324 [INCOMPLETE]

Tampa, FL 33602
500 East Zack Street, Suite 610
813-273-4566

Washington, DC 20535
601 4th Street Northwest
202-278-2000

FEDERAL, STATE, AND TERRITORIAL HEALTHCARE AUTHORITIES

Federal Authorities

Domestic Preparedness Helpline (Monday through Friday, 0900 to 1800)
800-368-6498

CDC Emergency Preparedness and Response Branch
770-488-7100

National Response Center
800-424-8802

U.S. Army MRIID
888-872-7443 (800-USA-RIID)

U.S. Public Health Service (PHS)
800-872-6367

Bioport Corporation (anthrax vaccine manufacturer)
Lansing, MI 48906
517-327-1500

State and Territorial Authorities

Alabama
Department of Public Health
State Health Officer
334-206-5200
fax: 334-206-2008

Alaska
Division of Public Health
Director
907-465-3090
fax: 907-586-1877

American Samoa
Department of Health
Director
684-633-4606
fax: 684-633-5379

Arizona
Department of Health Services
Director
602-542-1025
fax: 602-542-1062

Arkansas
Department of Health
Director
501-661-2417
fax: 501-671-1450

California
Department of Health Services
State Health Officer
916-657-1493
fax: 916-657-3089

Colorado
Department of Public Health & Environment
Executive Director
303-692-2011
fax: 303-691-7702

Connecticut
Department of Public Health
Commissioner
860-509-7101
fax: 860-509-7111

Delaware
Division of Public Health
Director
302-739-4700
fax: 302-739-6659

District of Columbia
Department of Health
Acting Director
202-645-5556
fax: 202-645-0526

Florida
Department of Health
Secretary and State Health Officer
850-487-2945
fax: 850-487-3729

Georgia
Division of Public Health
Director
404-657-2700
fax: 404-657-2715

Guam
Department of Public Health & Social Services
Director of Health
671-735-7102
fax: 671-734-5910

Hawaii
Department of Health
Director
808-586-4410
fax: 808-586-4444

Idaho
Division of Health
Administrator
208-334-5945
fax: 208-334-6581

Illinois
Department of Public Health
Director of Public Health
217-782-4977
fax: 217-782-3987

Indiana
Department of Health
State Health Commissioner
317-233-7400
fax: 317-233-7387

Iowa
Department of Public Health
Director of Public Health
515-281-5605
fax: 515-281-4958

Kansas
Department of Health and Environment
Director of Health
785-296-1343
fax: 785-296-1562

Kentucky
Department for Public Health
Commissioner
502-564-3970
fax: 502-564-6533

Louisiana
Department of Health and Hospitals
State Health Officer
504-342-8093
fax: 504-342-8098

Maine
Bureau of Health
Director
207-287-3201
fax: 207-287-4631

Mariana Islands
Department of Public Health & Environmental Services
Secretary of Health and Environmental Services
670-234-8950
fax: 670-234-8930

Marshall Islands
Majuro Hospital
Minister of Health & Environmental Services
692-625-3355
fax: 692-625-3432

Maryland
Department of Health and Mental Hygiene
Secretary
410-767-6505
fax: 410-767-6489

Massachusetts
Department of Public Health
Commissioner
617-624-5200
fax: 617-624-5206

Michigan
Community Public Health Agency
Chief Executive and Medical Officer
517-335-8024
fax: 517-335-9476

Micronesia
Department of Health Services
Secretary of Health
691-320-2619
fax: 691-320-5263

Minnesota
Department of Health
Commissioner of Health
651-296-8401
fax: 651-215-5801

Mississippi
State Department of Health
State Health Officer and Chief Executive
601-960-7634
fax: 601-960-7931

Missouri
Department of Health
Director
573-751-6001
fax: 573-751-6041

Montana
Department of Public Health & Human Services
Director
406-444-5622
fax: 406-444-1970

Nebraska
Health and Human Services System
Chief Medical Officer
402-471-8399
fax: 402-471-9449

Nevada
Division of Health
Health Officer
702-687-3786
fax: 702-687-3859

New Hampshire
Department of Health & Human Services
Medical Director
603-271-4372
fax: 603-271-4827

New Jersey
Department of Health & Senior Services
Commissioner of Health
609-292-7837
fax: 609-292-0053

New Mexico
Department of Health
Secretary
505-827-2613
fax: 505-827-2530

New York
State Department of Health
Commissioner of Health
518-474-2011
fax: 518-474-5450

North Carolina
Department of Health and Human Services
State Health Director
919-733-4392
fax: 919-715-4645

North Dakota
Department of Health
State Health Officer
701-328-2372
fax: 701-328-4727

Ohio
Department of Health
Director of Health
614-466-2253
fax: 614-644-0085

Oklahoma
Department of Health
Commissioner of Health
405-271-4200
fax: 405-271-3431

Oregon
Health Division
Administrator
503-731-4000
fax: 503-731-4078

Palau, Republic of
Ministry of Health
Minister of Health
680-488-2813
fax: 680-488-1211

Pennsylvania
Department of Health
Secretary of Health
717-787-6436
fax: 717-787-0191

Puerto Rico
Department of Health
Secretary of Health
787-274-7602
fax: 787-250-6547

Rhode Island
Department of Health
Director of Health
401-277-2231
fax: 401-277-6548

South Carolina
Department of Health and Environmental Control
Commissioner
803-734-4880
fax: 803-734-4620

South Dakota
Department of Health
Secretary of Health
605-773-3361
fax: 605-773-5683

Tennessee
Department of Health
State Health Officer
615-741-3111
fax: 615-741-2491

Texas
Department of Health
Commissioner of Health
512-458-7375
fax: 512-458-7477

Utah
Department of Health
Director
801-538-6111
fax: 801-538-6306

Vermont

Department of Health
Commissioner
802-863-7280
fax: 802-865-7754

Virgin Islands

Department of Health
Commissioner of Health
340-774-0117
fax: 340-777-4001

Virginia

Department of Health
State Health Commissioner
804-786-3561
fax: 804-786-4616

Washington

State Department of Health
Acting Secretary of Health
360-753-5871
fax: 360-586-7424

West Virginia

Bureau for Public Health
Commissioner of Health
304-558-2971
fax: 304-558-1035

Wisconsin

Department of Health and Family Services
Administrator
608-266-1511
fax: 608-267-2832

Wyoming

Department of Health
Director
307-777-7656
fax: 307-777-7439

INDEX